Circuits
for the
MRCPCH

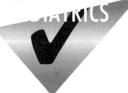

PAEDIATRICS

Dedication
To Gaggy who, in his own way, inspired.

Commissioning Editor: Ellen Green, Pauline Graham
Development Editor: Clive Hewat
Project Manager: Christine Johnston
Design Direction: Erik Bigland
Illustration Manager: Gillian Richards
Illustrator: Barking Dog Art

Circuits
for the
MRCPCH

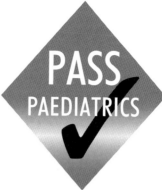

Damian Roland BMBS BMedSci MRCPCH

Paediatric Specialist Registrar and Honorary University Fellow
Peninsula Medical School
Plymouth, UK

Richard Neal MA MB BChir MRCPCH

Paediatric Specialist Registrar
Lincoln County Hospital
Lincoln, UK

Shabna Rajapaksa MA MB BChir MRCPCH

Paediatric Specialist Registrar
Royal Berkshire Hospital
Reading, UK

FOREWORD BY
Terence Stephenson BSc BM BCh DM FRCP FRCPCH

Professor of Child Health and Dean of the Faculty
Medicine and Health Sciences
The University of Nottingham
Nottingham, UK

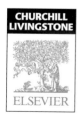

EDINBURGH LONDON NEW YORK OXFORD PHILADELPHIA ST LOUIS SYDNEY
TORONTO 2007

ELSEVIER
CHURCHILL
LIVINGSTONE

© 2007, Elsevier Limited. All rights reserved.

The right of Damian Roland to be identified as editor of this work has been asserted by him in accordance with the Copyright, Designs and Patents Act 1988.

ISBN 978 0 443 10335 3

British Library Cataloguing in Publication Data
A catalogue record for this book is available from the British Library

Library of Congress Cataloging in Publication Data
A catalog record for this book is available from the Library of Congress

Note
Knowledge and best practice in this field are constantly changing. As new research and experience broaden our knowledge, changes in practice, treatment and drug therapy may become necessary or appropriate. Readers are advised to check the most current information provided (i) on procedures featured or (ii) by the manufacturer of each product to be administered, to verify the recommended dose or formula, the method and duration of administration, and contraindications. It is the responsibility of the practitioner, relying on their own experience and knowledge of the patient, to make diagnoses, to determine dosages and the best treatment for each individual patient, and to take all appropriate safety precautions. To the fullest extent of the law, neither the Publisher nor the Editor assumes any liability for any injury and/or damage to persons or property arising out of or related to any use of the material contained in this book.

The Publisher

Working together to grow
libraries in developing countries

www.elsevier.com | www.bookaid.org | www.sabre.org

ELSEVIER   BOOK AID
International   Sabre Foundation

your source for books,
journals and multimedia
in the health sciences

www.elsevierhealth.com

The
Publisher's
policy is to use
**paper manufactured
from sustainable forests**

Printed in China

Contents

Foreword

Damian Roland and his colleagues have written a truly excellent book. As someone who has tried to write books to guide previous generations of trainees through MRCPCH exams, I know that what the reader wants is a book written by someone who has sat the exam themselves, passed the exam and can provide real insights into the conduct of the exam. They want a book written in an easily readable style and ideally to show sympathy and humour as well as provide information. This book ticks all those boxes.

The previous version of the MRCPCH exam, like many of the professional exams run by the Royal Colleges, gave rise to a fund of stories, no doubt many apocryphal, relating to both the exam cases and the examiners. The clinical exam was often viewed as something of a lottery, almost entirely dependent on which cases the candidate saw and whether the child (or indeed the parent) was in a good mood or not. There were allegations that examiners asked questions only on their favourite topics and that the examiners themselves could not elicit the physical signs that they were asking the candidate to elicit. Some examiners were thought to be particularly dyspeptic after a parsimonious lunch provided by the cash-strapped local NHS hospital running the exam. They longed for the halcyon days of examiners' dinners and fine wines!

The new format of the MRCPCH examination has been developed to try and address many of these concerns. Fundamentally, a postgraduate professional exam should examine trainees in the things they need to know. Therefore, the keystones remain history-taking, examination of physical signs, clinical skills and, very importantly, communication, both with the child and their family. The circuit exam sets out to do this but brings the benefits of being robust, reproducible and, as far as possible, equitable to all the candidates attending on any one day. As someone who has examined both the old format and the new format, I believe that the new format is fairer to candidates if rather more boring for the examiners!

I would strongly recommend that you read, learn and inwardly digest the material within this book. It is written from the heart and it is written with your interests in mind. I am sure it will assist you in your aspiration to be a fully trained and competent paediatrician because, while the advice is geared to helping you pass the MRCPCH exam, the advice is also about good practice in taking histories, examining children and communicating.

Professor Terence Stephenson
Nottingham, 2007

Acknowledgements

This book would not have been possible without the input of Dr Laura Hole, Dr Simon Robinson, Dr Elizabeth Evans – or without the help of Dr Craig Sayers and Dr Alex Allwood and most importantly the patience of Miss Katie Borlase.

Introduction

If you have not already done so, stand up and give yourself a big hug. Congratulations! You have managed to stand the pressure, heartache and pain of two of the hardest exams you will ever sit. The written exams are over; no more ambiguous questions, no more basic science, and no more exam halls. Be proud of yourself; there is but one more hurdle …

The clinical component of the MRCPCH was entirely revamped for October 2004 in an effort to become more accountable to the educationalists, be fairer on candidates and change the emphasis of the exam. It has now been running for 2 years and used as a tool to assess aspiring SHOs against the standard of a first-year specialist registrar. This is an important change as you are now being graded against a specific objective. By the time you take the exam you should be fed up with baby checks and reviewing erythema toxicum. You should want to be in clinic seeing new patients rather than writing up paracetamol. You want to be the first person the nurses call when the really sick child arrives. Passing the exam is the gateway to all of those things.

This book is written with an important underlying principle. It is not a textbook of definitive fact and differential lists. It will not take you step by step through a thorough neurological exam. And it will not help you pass if you have no background knowledge! This textbook has been written by people who have taken the exam while it is still fresh in their minds. It has been written by candidates who know how hard examiners can make things for you. It has been written by junior doctors who, like yourselves, had no idea what to expect but went on to pass the exam. The circuits presented contain the questions and scenarios you will encounter. They contain the experiences and advice of candidates who each had different approaches and styles but used common principles to reach the same objective – the pass mark.

It would be very easy to start reading through the circuits now and I have often skipped through the seeming waffle at the front of many textbooks. However, I would really recommend reading through the 'How to get the most out of this book' section. It contains useful information on exam strategy, revision optimisation and, most importantly, getting the most out of the questions. You may well get frustrated with this book if you don't!

Best wishes for the exam,

Damian Roland

Note: The term SHO is used for those below middle grade. With the advent of Modernising Medical careers it is likely that scenarios involving F1 and F2 will eventually become more common. However, this does not change the way these questions are approached.

HOW TO GET THE MOST OUT OF THIS BOOK

The prototype circuit is shown below and this should be well known to you, as should all the information on the College website (*www.rcpch. ac.uk*). You should study the website as not only does it explain the circuit in great detail but also it will keep you up to date on any subtle changes. Example questions can be found by going to the website, selecting 'Publications' and then clicking on 'Publications Section'. An alphabetical list will be shown; click on 'Examinations' and you will be given all documentation pertaining to all three membership exams. You will find example questions as well as information for candidates and examiners (both worth looking at).

Essentially the exam consists of ten stations: six involving patient interaction (clinical), two communication role-play, a history-taking and management planning station and a video station showing acute signs and symptoms. The latter station does not lend itself well to revision by book so is not covered any further. There is an example CD available from the College to let you know what it's about.

The basic examination circuit is represented in the diagram below:

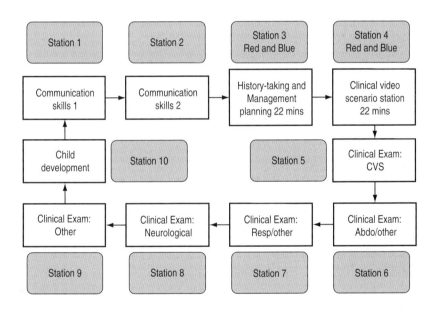

- 1 examiner per station, none for clinical video scenario stations.
- 10 examiners for the circuit, 1 additional examiner for back-up/quality assurance.
- Candidates join at each station of the circuit, making 12 in total per circuit.
- 2 candidates join at the History taking and Management planning stations and 2 at the Clinical video scena station at any one time.
- In total there are 10 objective assessments per candidate.
- The History-taking and Management planning stations and the Clinical video scenario stations are 22 minutes in length, with the other 8 stations being of 9 minutes' duration.
- There are 4-minute breaks between each station, with the entire circuit taking 152 minutes to complete.
- The sequence in which a candidate takes the stations in the circuit will vary.

Royal College of Paediatrics and Child Health, October 2004. MRCPCH Clinical Examination
www.repch.ac.uk/publications/examinations_documents/Web_Circuit.pdf

Each station is 9 minutes long, except the history-taking and management planning station, which lasts 22 minutes. In the exam the 9 minutes seem to disappear as quickly as butter on a hot day so you must be swift (but not rushed) in the clinical stations. Of the six clinical stations, cardiology, neurology and development must be covered. There is generic advice that two of the other three stations should be respiratory and abdominal but this is not an absolute.

Each of the eight chapters is presented as an exam circuit without the video station. They are therefore divided up into nine stations and you will find that each commences with the wording you will get in the actual exam. This is essentially generic information about the type of station, how long it lasts and whether you are to have any supplementary material. For the clinical stations in the exam you will be told what the station is and then have to wait 4 minutes before being presented with your patient. Rather than just sit there and dwell over the last station you feel you failed, I suggest you start thinking through your examination for the station to come. Obviously you can't do this for the 'other' stations but cardiology and neurology stations must have those systems to examine. For the clinical stations, beneath the generic blurb is the examiner's request, the description of the child you are to examine and potentially some further questions on what you might do next. Please bear in mind the following points:

1. At first read-through the book may appear a bit 'wordy'. A lot of the detail in the answer sections is actually based around the exam process rather than hard fact. Much of this needn't be read in detail second time round as they are easy points to learn. The key clinical information will be found in highlighted tables and boxes.
2. The scenarios may appear vague in places. The aim is not to deliberately confuse but to recreate some of the dilemmas you actually have in the exam. No situation in medicine is ever black and white. Unlike previous revision texts there are few classic cases in this book. Too often candidates learn ideal descriptions of pathology or syndromes but when presented with the case in the exam they either don't actually recognize those features – e.g. what does a shagreen patch look like in tuberous sclerosis? – or they don't have the features you think they should (only 15% of those with neurofibromatosis have optic glioma). Before looking at the answer to the question write down a list of differentials. How much do you know about each of the conditions on that list?
3. The book contains very few pictures. The reason is that there are not many good pictures available on the public domain and most are already used in paediatric textbooks. These conditions are easy to recognise and don't represent the children you will have in the exam. Obviously text cannot replace actually seeing the child in question but it will focus your mind on the important features to look for.
4. Before looking at the answer make sure you go through in your head all the questions you would have asked the parent/patient or which systems you would have examined more closely. You will be lulled into

a false sense of security if you read a question, spend 10 seconds thinking about your response and then look at the answers.

5. An answer is given for the clinical stations. However, it may not always have been possible to get that answer from the information given. This is to avoid classic scenarios being given which do not encourage active thought. The answer is provided to help when rereading chapters to quickly refresh your memory about the learning points of the station.

6. The answers are designed to direct further revision. They will present a structure to answering the station and provide helpful hints about that particular condition. In some cases they will give you a definitive conclusion as to the case but, as you will discover in the exam, you do not necessarily have to be spot on to pass the station. Nor does getting the right diagnosis mean you have fulfilled the examiner's instructions.

7. No apology is made for the occasional repetition of information or similarity between some stations. In researching this book it has become obvious that certain information and themes pop up all too frequently.

8. When you start getting annoyed that the information given is lacking in places and the answer isn't definite because you know of confounding issues, then you are ready to take the exam!

The communication and history-taking stations are slightly different from the clinical ones as, just as in the examination, you are given a scenario to look through before the station starts. This sets the scene, gives you your role and provides information on the patient/parent/family you will be talking to. As you are given a maximum of 2 minutes' reading time it will be worth doing at least some of these questions with a stopwatch to create exam conditions.

At the end of some of the questions there may be summary boxes recapping the important information that needs to have been gleaned for that particular station. The 'Can you?' box literally just asks if you can recap the points implied in the question. For quick revision sessions these can be directly referred to if you have a spare 5 minutes.

You will find there is more generic descriptive advice in the earlier chapters, changing to more detailed clinical fact as the book progresses. This is to avoid repetition of learning points, although important issues will be re-emphasised.

Below is some general advice for each of the stations in the circuits. It is worth reading this before looking at the first chapter. From then on there is no set way to proceed. Individually it can be used chapter by chapter to ensure you are covering the important points and are not missing key information. The first couple of chapters may be used as you start revising to give you direction. You may return to the book later to check your progress. In groups the chapters will facilitate discussion about topics and will provide a large amount of scope for practice role-play. It is hoped clinicians who have membership but have not taken the new exam will use it to aid their own teaching. I would also recommend watching *House* or renting previous series on DVD. The medicine is very silly but almost every episode requires you to come up with a differential for presenting symptoms. Of course these are either often adults, exceedingly rare or a result of House's own treatment! They do require you to think on the spot, though. Do not go into the exam having never been challenged to produce a list of differentials on the spur of the moment.

I hope this book will be a valuable learning aid and help to ease some of the tension on what may be the last exam of your life!

CARDIOLOGY

Cardiology and neurology short cases are now essential parts of the circuit. There is no excuse for not having prepared yourself for the identification and classification of heart murmurs. The old maxim, 'Common things are common', is noted well here. The College has made clear they would like to see the newly qualified registrar examined on things they are likely to see. With ventriculoseptal defect (VSD) being the most common congenital cardiac anomaly, these (one would hope) will be the murmurs you are likely to hear. Unfortunately the exam is not a test of your applied knowledge of epidemiology; it is much less forgiving …

Generally candidates are good at picking up systolic murmurs and being able to give an approximate location. They are more nervous about diastolic murmurs and the presence of thrills. Much like all of clinical medicine, the more you do/see the better you get. Unlike syndromes, from which you may make a diagnosis having actually only ever seen a picture in a book, it is difficult to do this with cardiology. It is vital, for example, that you have seen a VSD with a thrill and know how to differentiate this from other systolic murmurs. Cardiology clinics are a good place to do this but some candidates may want to go on a course – which in the author's opinion is money well spent.

Confident presentation is important in all parts of the exam but can be especially difficult because the examiner knows what the murmur is, and you are either right or wrong. On close questioning the candidates may be tempted to change their diagnosis three or four times on the basis of a raised eyebrow! Unfortunately there are few 'soft' signs; you need to know your AS from your PS and not get ADD about ASD*. Importantly, your examination findings must tally with your diagnosis. The examiner will forgive you for missing the inconsequential tricuspid regurgitation but not if you tell him a systolic murmur at the left sternal edge is mitral stenosis. It is generally accepted that it is wiser to leave the diagnosis until you have presented your findings. One of the authors opted for the converse approach and was fortunately right, although he spent the rest of the 9 minutes answering difficult questions – perhaps best to waste time talking!

If you still have the box from your Littmann stethoscope you may find a CD of common heart murmurs in it – or try *www.dartmouth.edu/~clipp/demo_case.htm* and log on as a guest for a very good cardiology-type station.

---

*As, aortic stenosis; PS, pulmonary stenosis; ADD, attention deficit disorder; ASD, atrial septal defects.

ABDO/RESPIRATORY/OTHER

Without going into the realms of specific examination there is honestly little new to say with regard to these stations apart from the fact that practice makes perfect! They are classic short cases and should be treated as such. You are given 4 minutes' preparation time before the station, and although the station may be 'other', the time is well spent rehearsing your examination flow and reminding yourself of differential lists. By the time you have walked into the room, had the story explained, introduced yourself and positioned the patient you will be well into your 9 minutes of time. It will go quickly so make sure the exam is precise but slick. It is therefore important you know how long your examinations take you. You should be able to perform a good abdominal or respiratory exam in a couple of minutes. If you are taking 5 minutes the examiner will get bored and stop you. It is very useful to watch other candidates examining but all too easy to criticise other people's techniques. Feedback is vital from registrars who have passed the exam.

NEUROLOGY

As will be repeated later in the book there is no excuse for not knowing your neurological exam inside out. Yes, it can be the most difficult of the clinical stations and, yes, it can be the most difficult to get good feedback and teaching on. However, you will be examined on it so there is no point in putting your head in the sand. The problem for some candidates is, despite knowing how to perform the 'perfect' exam, the application and interpretation of the results are still difficult. Candidates easily get distracted from their routine because they are concerned about getting the whole answer rather than the specific sign in question. Have senior physicians examine you and stop you randomly during the exam to ask you what you have found (this can be applied to all exams; it keeps you on your toes and makes sure you are listening, feeling, etc.!).

Most difficult is guessing what the examiner would like you to do. Diagnosis of neurological conditions demands you are able to quickly assess an area and accurately examine subsequent body parts/function with a differential in mind. You should then be able to predict what other features may be present to confirm your diagnosis – all very difficult in 9 minutes and in the stress of the exam!

Registrars can teach most clinical examinations – even those who have only recently passed MRCPCH. However, specialists should teach precise neurological exam. Generally, looking technically confident and being swift but precise are the hardest skills to master.

DEVELOPMENT

For many candidates who sit the exam this station is the greatest unknown. A simple idea in theory, it is one of the most difficult to revise for. Obviously a sound knowledge of developmental milestones is necessary but the skill is in the interpretation and testing of them. You may be able to say a 2-year-old has not reached his milestones but do you know why? Do you know where he is at the moment? Is his apparent deficit a result of another delayed milestone?

Interestingly, although it may seem hard to find practice cases, potentially every child seen on the ward can be used. Examining fellow candidates about normality, especially the written and verbal components, will be especially helpful for isolated delays. Those who have worked in the community obviously have some advantage, but remember the test is devised for those without specific developmental experience. Make sure you know normal and the variations thereof. Ask to spend a morning at the hospital nursery walking through from the infants, to the toddlers and then the pre-schoolers. You will see a wide range of development in children who are the same age but have no special needs.

A familiarity with the tools necessary to assess development is useful. These include balls, cubes and drawing implements. Make sure you have interacted with a child to get them to make various objects, etc. The heat of the exam is not the time to discover you can't make a four-block tower yourself!

COMMUNICATION

The College is proud of its communication skills stations, in part because they bring it into line with fashionable educationalist medicine but also because it is a generally fair and good discriminator. Like or loathe 'role-play', it has become central to medical education and most candidates should have experienced it during their university training. The ability to get into the 'spirit' of the exercise will help determine the outcome to a great extent. Don't forget though that you should be doing things you have done before. It is apparent to the examiner when you are unfamiliar with a particular approach. Take breaking the news to a mother that her child needs some further investigation for a possible blood malignancy. It is possible you may not have done this specific task in a real clinical setting. However, you should have at least observed this taking place or broken news in a similar vein. One might argue if you are not confident about this it might be worth delaying the exam in order to gain this skill. Even if you are confident, has anyone observed you doing this? Have you received feedback about your communication skills? (nurses are a valuable resource in this regard). Candidates often realise they have quite funny mannerisms and gestures when talking (and also presenting, so not just specific to this station). Some of these may be manipulated with practice. Make sure you don't look even more uncomfortable by placing your expressive hands behind your back though!

This station is easily practised with colleagues so make sure you are well prepared, especially with the 'difficult' patient. Placating an angry adult is not an easy skill and the College has made no secret of the fact it may use actors to do this. Remember that communication may also be between health care professionals, including nurses, doctors and medical students.

The following question is an example station taken from the College website.

CANDIDATE INFORMATION

This station assesses your ability to deal with a clinical problem.

This is a 9-minute station consisting of spoken interaction. You will have up to 2 minutes before the start of the station to read this sheet and prepare yourself. You may make notes on the paper provided.

When the bell sounds you will be invited into the examination room. Please take this instruction sheet with you. The examiner will not ask questions during the 9 minutes but will warn you when you have approximately 2 minutes left.

You are not required to examine a patient.

The encounter should be focused on the task; you will be penalised for asking irrelevant questions or providing superfluous information. You will be marked on your ability to communicate, not the speed with which you convey information. You may not have time to complete the communication.

You are: An SpR in paediatrics.

Setting: Side room of paediatric ward during a Sunday morning ward round.

You will be talking to: Sally Jones, the mother of David Jones, a 5-week-old baby who was born at term, birth weight 3.5 kg. You have not previously been involved in this baby's care.

Background: David is being investigated for prolonged conjugated jaundice. During the night David has become drowsy and is not feeding and has been having brief periods of apnoea and is requiring supplemental oxygen to maintain his saturations at more than 90%.

You have noted that David was meant to have been prescribed phenobarbital (phenobarbitone) 15 mg once a day, 2 days previously but instead has been given 75 mg once daily as the writing on the prescription was misinterpreted.

His jaundice started on the second day of life. He was given phototherapy treatment in hospital for days 2–5 but has been jaundiced ever since. He was initially breast-fed but his mother's milk dried up.

> **Task: To talk to Mrs Jones about the prescribing error and its effects on her son.**

YOU ARE NOT EXPECTED TO GATHER THE REST OF THE MEDICAL HISTORY DURING THIS CONSULTATION.

MRCPCH COMMUNICATION SKILLS STATION

ROLE-PLAYER INFORMATION

This is a 9-minute station, consisting of spoken interaction between you and the candidate. There is no discussion with the examiner.

You are: Sally Jones, the mother of David Jones, a 5-week-old baby being investigated for prolonged jaundice. This started on the second day of life. He was given phototherapy (fluorescent light) treatment in hospital for days 2–5 but has been jaundiced ever since. You took him home 1 week after birth.

You breast-fed him for 2 weeks but your milk dried up.

He has been started on a drug as part of his investigations but unfortunately has been given five times the intended dose.

David is your first child. His current admission to hospital has been for 2 days. You have noticed that he is very sleepy.

David has not eaten today. He is jaundiced and has stopped breathing briefly. He is currently receiving oxygen via a tube under his nose and is on a saturation monitor.

Your general feelings:

- You show controlled anger.
- You want to know why this has happened.

After the doctor has explained the situation to you, your feelings and further questions are:

- Why is he now on oxygen?
- What are the potential problems/side effects?
- Will it delay the investigations for his jaundice?
- What will be done by the hospital to prevent it happening again?

What to expect from the candidate, and how to respond:

- Offer an apology.
- An explanation of the hospital's complaints procedure.

The main thing is to be CONSISTENT with your story and emotional response with each candidate.

This station assesses the candidate's ability to deal with a clinical problem.

This is a 9-minute station consisting of spoken interaction between the candidate and the role-player. You should remind the candidate when 2 minutes remain otherwise you should remain silent during the examination time.

If the candidate finishes early, you should check that they have finished. If yes, they should remain in the room until the session has ended.

INFORMATION GIVEN TO CANDIDATE:

You are: An SpR in paediatrics.

Setting: Side room of paediatric ward during a Sunday morning ward round.

You will be talking to: Sally Jones, the mother of David Jones, a 5-week-old baby who was born at term, birth weight 3.5 kg. You have not previously been involved in this baby's care.

Background: David is being investigated for prolonged conjugated jaundice. During the night David has become drowsy and is not feeding and has been having brief periods of apnoea and is requiring supplemental oxygen to maintain his saturations at more than 90%.

You have noted that David was meant to have been prescribed phenobarbital (phenobarbitone) 15 mg once a day, 2 days previously but instead has been given 75 mg once daily as the writing on the prescription was misinterpreted.

His jaundice started on the second day of life. He was given phototherapy treatment in hospital for days 2–5 but has been jaundiced ever since. He was initially breast-fed but his mother's milk dried up.

> **Task:** To talk to Mrs Jones about the prescribing error and its effects on her son.

INFORMATION GIVEN TO ROLE-PLAYER:

You are: Sally Jones, the mother of David Jones, a 5-week-old baby being investigated for prolonged jaundice. This started on the second day of life. He was given phototherapy (fluorescent lights) treatment in hospital for days 2–5 but has been jaundiced ever since. You took him home 1 week after birth.

You breast-fed him for 2 weeks but your milk dried up.

He has been started on a drug as part of his investigations but unfortunately has been given five times the intended dose.

David is your first child. His current admission to hospital has been for 2 days. You have noticed that he is very sleepy.

MRCPCH COMMUNICATION SKILLS STATION

EXAMINER INFORMATION (page one)

David has not eaten today. He is jaundiced and has stopped breathing briefly. He is currently receiving oxygen via a tube under his nose and is on a saturation monitor.

Your general feelings:

- You show controlled anger.
- You want to know why this has happened.

GUIDE NOTES TOWARDS EXPECTED STANDARD:

- Appropriate conduct of interview.
- An explanation to the parents of how the error occurred.
- To apologise for the reported mistake.
- To recap the situation and to invite parents' questions about the possible toxic effects to David and how these will be monitored.
- To detail the actions necessary which will include:
  - notification of an adverse incident to the Hospital Trust.
  - to document fully in the medical records of the patient the prescribing error and actions taken.
- Closure – reassurance, final apology.

EXAMINER INFORMATION (page two)

Please use this sheet to make a list of the criteria you have used in this station to decide if a candidate is a clear pass, pass, bare fail or clear fail and hand it to the host examiner when you have completed the circuit.

CLEAR PASS ...

PASS ...

BARE FAIL ...

CLEAR FAIL ...

Note that one of the key points to achieve, other than an adequate explanation, the ability to apologise and good communication skills, was that you would complete an incident form. The communications skills station not only assesses basic rapport but also assumes sound clinical knowledge and risk management skills.

The communication stations are very open ended, with the nature of the ground to be explored dependent on the actor/patient employed. Parents may be angry, over-anxious, not well informed or perhaps misinformed. The actual guidelines for the role-player are very loosely worded, so that no two stations on the same day will be the same.

You will see you are assumed to have a thorough understanding of the medical issues involved for the children in these stations. If you are asked questions you do not know the answer to it is vital that you do not make things up or be hesitant. There is no reason why you cannot say you will seek advice on this issue from your consultant (although if you are deferring every question you may find it difficult to pass!).

HISTORY-TAKING/MANAGEMENT PLANNING

It is beyond the remit of this book to teach history-taking and the management of complex or rare chronic conditions. Like the communication skills stations, there are consistently familiar themes to the approach of these scenarios. It is good practice to jot down a few pointers while waiting for the station to begin that will direct your questions. This is not an easy station and the fact that you take histories every day in the admissions unit is not the same as the outpatient-focused history. It is easy to get distracted by taking every possible detail at the expense of information which will help your management plan. It is also difficult (and some would say unnatural) to only take a history and not to explain and clarify certain information to the child's parents.

Make time to be observed taking a focused history of a new referral to an outpatient clinic to a consultant or senior registrar (this may well be difficult to organise). It is amazing when being observed how under pressure you feel and what simple things you forget to ask. Remember this is management planning in a non-acute scenario. Simply requesting bloods is unlikely to be the answer. Referral to other centres and disciplines is likely to be a useful process; remember you are acting as a first-year registrar.

Clinic experience is essential to understanding the process behind these stations.

USEFUL REVISION WEBSITES

www.virtualpediatrichospital.org good generic information with many practice scenarios

www.pediatriceducation.org the cases are useful for communication and history and management planning stations

PLAYING THE GAME

The clinical exam requires the same expert understanding of paediatrics and child health as the previous two written papers. It also adds in the unpredictable element of the examiner. Many candidates, despite feeling they had the skills and knowledge to pass, blame the unnecessarily difficult professor on their failure. Stories of 'hawks' reducing candidates to tears are recounted by SHOs, registrars and the consultants themselves. Even those candidates who pass will often wax lyrical about the battle they had with the obstinate examiner over the station that nearly failed them. This indicates that some of the bitterness generated isn't always related to sour grapes at failing the exam (although this can certainly be the case if candidates are honest with themselves).

There is something distinctly unusual about having your every word and movement monitored. Just this act of observation can reduce good trainee paediatricians to the level of a newly qualified foundation grade. The only other time you are observed in this way, with so much pressure riding on the result, is medical finals and your driving test. I am no longer ashamed to say that I passed my driving test on my seventh – yes seventh, attempt. At the time I was the laughing stock of my peers – a seemingly intelligent, motivated and able sixth-form student cracking under the pressure of a three-point turn. In hindsight there were a few reasons why this occurred. I failed my first test with a D (dangerous driving!) as a result of just not being ready for the exam. I was practically much improved on the second attempt but I had this nagging doubt in my mind. Most of my peers passed first time or, at the worst, second time round. What would happen if I failed? With that small seed planted I spent most of the test paranoid that every little mistake I made was being held against me. At one stage I thought I had pulled out in front of someone and glimpsed the examiner placing a cross on his sheet. I was furious, stopped concentrating and then made a string of small but costly errors. In fact I had not failed for my initial mistake, and had I not got so distracted by this I probably would have passed. Unfortunately my obsession with what the examiner was doing resulted in failures in tests 3, 4, 5 and 6 as well. There are numerous lessons to be learnt here:

1. Don't let me drive you anywhere.
2. Do not sit the exam until you are ready. You must seek an honest opinion from a senior colleague who knows you well and has seen you examine patients. You are doing yourself no favours by failing badly on your first attempt. It will damage your confidence and you lose the benefit of having taken the exam early to speed up your time through the system.
3. You must learn to stop thinking about the examiner and concentrate on the patient. Be truly interested in diagnosing the condition the child has. This sounds cheesy but unless you are focusing all your efforts on the child then you are wasting the knowledge and time you have spent getting to the exam.
4. You have not failed until the College sends you a letter telling you, 'You've failed!'. I realise this is flippant but there is no point spending £300 to give up after two stations because you feel it is all over.
5. Although the college won't let you take the exam seven times in a row, if you truly believe in yourself you stand a much better chance of passing. I have seen candidates go into the exam with that seed of doubt already planted; it will sprout very quickly in the heat of the exam circuit.

There are a few classic tips that you should be aware of by now. I apologise for potentially preaching to the converted but the little things do matter. Some of these points are repeated in different guises at later points in the book to ensure you are listening!

Examine someone else in a pressure situation. The best candidate is actually a medical student preparing for (paediatric) finals. This puts you in a position of clinical superiority. Place yourself in the examiner's shoes and examine a child who has, in your opinion, an obvious clinical sign. You do not have to be unnecessarily harsh or unkind but make sure the student has approached the patient in a professional manner, examined diligently, picked up the sign and answered some of your questions about aetiology or management. Afterwards ask your candidate about their thoughts and feelings about you. You may find you made them nervous by your very presence. What were your questions like? Did you come across as friendly or mean? It is likely that the examiner role will cast you in a light you are not comfortable with. Many examiners say they do their level best to help but the candidates seem to be able to dig their own holes!

Dress well and look the part. This means:

- Wear glasses as opposed to contacts if you are not sure which to wear.
- Don't wear a ridiculous tie unless you have a consistent personality to match. Ask senior physicians if you come across as too flamboyant or too quiet.

- Be videoed at least once examining a real or mock patient. Watch yourself. Are there any mannerisms you have which you need to alter? Do you speak too quickly? Are you as clear in your pronunciation as you thought?

Be prepared for the question, 'Are you sure?'. The examiner will ask this question for two reasons and two reasons alone. It is not because they are trying to trick you.

- *You look like you are not sure.* If you spend 3 minutes listening to the same spot on the precordium or ask the child to walk seven times across the room, you simply do not look confident. If you do not have a definitive answer simply describe what you have seen or heard. You can then give your most likely differentials. Remember, not all the children in the exam need to be given a diagnosis to pass.
- *You have provided inconsistent information.* 'This pink and well-perfused 7-year-old child has a loud murmur at the left sternal edge. There are no scars to see. This child may have a VSD or Fallot's tetralogy.' Stupid example but it is very easy to say things under pressure. The examiners understand this and just want to make sure you don't actually mean what you have just said.

The key to passing some stations is to have the children on your side. Some of these kids have been coming to exam for years and have seen countless candidates excel or exterminate themselves. Introduce yourself to the child before their parent if they are over 5 years old. You may well find they appreciate the gesture.

Make sure you are comfortable with the normal size of children from 6 months to 5 years. If you are told a child is 3 years old you should be able to comment on whether their weight or height appears compatible with that. The examiners will expect you to be able to spot the malnourished or underdeveloped child and ask to see their weight and height charts.

Circuit A

This station assesses your ability to elicit clinical signs:
- **CVS**

This is a 9-minute station of clinical interaction. You will have up to 4 minutes beforehand to prepare yourself. No additional information will be given or is necessary before commencing the station. When the bell sounds you will be invited into the examination room.

INTRODUCTION

The examiner introduces you to Hannah, who is a 12-month-old girl. You are told that she spent the initial few months of her life in hospital and you are invited to examine her cardiovascular system.

CLINICAL SCENARIO

Hannah sits on her mother's lap without any oxygen therapy and is not dyspnoeic at rest. You are surprised she is 12 months old as she looks small for her age. Her head appears narrow when viewed face on and a little long in the anteroposterior direction. You ask the mother to remove her T-shirt. As you approach Hannah she begins to cry. You attempt to console her with the small teddy bear attached to your stethoscope. This makes matters worse. You notice that she has multiple small scars on her hands and a small scar on the left side of her chest.

You do manage to feel strong peripheral pulses and there is no evidence of central cyanosis. Useful examination of the chest and precordium is impossible due to Hannah's crying.

The examiner then asks you to comment on your findings thus far. What do you say?

This station assesses your ability to elicit clinical signs:
- Abdo/Other

This is a 9-minute station of clinical interaction. You will have up to 4 minutes beforehand to prepare yourself. No additional information will be given or is necessary before commencing the station. When the bell sounds you will be invited into the examination room.

INTRODUCTION

On entering the room you are told, 'This is Simon, who is a 16-year-old boy. Please examine his abdomen'.

CLINICAL SCENARIO

On inspection Simon is a thin boy and seems short for his age. He is pale and has a full and plethoric face. Despite his neck and shoulder blades having generous amounts of adipose tissue his extremities look wasted in comparison.

There are no peripheral stigmata of liver disease. He has three abdominal scars: two oblique scars in the left and right hypochondrium and one suprapubic scar. You also notice a small 2 cm scar close to his right clavicle. On palpation you find a left pelvic mass approximately 10 cm in length. It is non-tender, non-mobile and quite firm. He has no hepatosplenomegaly.

What do you think this pelvic mass is?

How do your clinical findings fit together?

What complications of treatment should be monitored?

STATION 3

This station assesses your ability to elicit clinical signs:

- **Neurological**

INTRODUCTION

The examiner says to you, 'This is Abdi. He is 11 years old and was born in Somalia. He was first treated by the ENT surgeons 5 years ago and since then his mother has been concerned about his face. Please examine his fifth, seventh and eighth cranial nerves using the equipment provided'.

CLINICAL SCENARIO

Abdi sits happily with his mother. On the table next to Abdi there is a piece of cotton wool and a tuning fork. At first glance there is a mild asymmetry to his face. You find no abnormality when you use the cotton wool to assess the sensation of the ophthalmic, maxillary and mandibular branches of the fifth cranial nerve. When you ask Abdi to screw up his eyes, puff out his cheeks and smile there is obvious weakness of the muscles in the left side of his face. He is unable to move his forehead on the left side. You place a vibrating tuning fork on the centre of the Abdi's head and ask him which side is louder. He tells you the left. You place the vibrating tuning fork next to his right ear and then place the base on the right mastoid process. He tells you it is louder when placed next to the ear. When repeated on the left side he tells you it is louder when placed on the bone, although you had difficulty finding the mastoid process due to scar tissue in this region.

Is there anything else you would like to examine?

How do you present your findings to the examiner?

What do you think may be the cause of these findings?

STATION 4

This station assesses your ability to elicit clinical signs:

- **Respiratory/Other**

This is a 9-minute station of clinical interaction. You will have up to 4 minutes beforehand to prepare yourself. No additional information will be given or is necessary before commencing the station. When the bell sounds you will be invited into the examination room.

INTRODUCTION

On entering the room the examiner says to you, 'This is Anthony, who is six. Have a look at his skin and then listen to his chest'.

CLINICAL SCENARIO

Anthony is an appropriate size for his age. On inspection of Anthony's skin you see he has dry, erythematous patches of skin covering his trunk, face and the flexor surfaces of his limbs. There are excoriated areas with visible scratch marks.

He is comfortable at rest and there is no evidence of cyanosis. There is no recession or indrawing. He is not barrel chested. You commence your exam by having a look at his hands. You notice no clubbing. The examiner stops you at this point and tells you he asked you to listen to his chest.

Auscultation of the chest is normal with no wheeze. The expiratory phase is normal.

You present your findings as a child with atopic eczema and a normal chest examination.

You are asked if he has Harrison's sulci. You are now concerned you are wrong but do not feel he has Harrison's sulci and he definitely does not have any wheeze.

What do you say to the examiner?

You are asked to explain to his mother how to manage the skin complaint. How would you do this?

STATION 5

This station assesses your ability to elicit clinical signs:
- **Other**

This is a 9-minute station of clinical interaction. You will have up to 4 minutes beforehand to prepare yourself. No additional information will be given or is necessary before commencing the station. When the bell sounds you will be invited into the examination room.

INTRODUCTION

On entering the room you are told, 'This is Nicola and her mother. Nicola is 7 years old. I'd like you to have a chat with her and ask her mum any questions you think may be important'.

CLINICAL SCENARIO

At first glance Nicola is a well-grown 7-year-old girl. Nicola talks throughout the examination with great enthusiasm about numerous subjects but with immaturity of content. You suspect she may have learning difficulty and have a good look for any dysmorphic features. She does not have Down's syndrome and you note blue eyes and small teeth for her age, although her lips are quite full and she has a slightly rounded end to her nose. As she talks it is apparent that she has below average intellect for an average 7-year-old.

What would you like to ask mum?

You are then asked to listen to her heart. She has a central sternotomy scar with keloid scarring. There are no other scars. Her heart sounds are normal.

How do these findings fit together?

What do you think the diagnosis is?

What else would you like to ask mum to aid your diagnosis in light of the cardiac abnormality?

This station assesses your ability to assess specifically requested areas in a child with a developmental problem:

- Development

This is a 9-minute station of clinical interaction. You will have up to 4 minutes beforehand to prepare yourself. No additional information will be given or is necessary before commencing the station. When the bell sounds you will be invited into the examination room.

INTRODUCTION

'This is Helen and her mother. Helen's mum was concerned about her speech development compared to other children. Before asking mother any questions what do you think of Helen's developmental age?'

CLINICAL SCENARIO

Helen is sitting at a table on your entrance to the room. She has been given some bricks to play with and she is currently hitting two of them together. She is suspicious of your arrival and looks between you and her mother. You introduce yourself to her mother and then to Helen. She says something incomprehensible to her mother, who smiles at her. You approach the table and ask her name. Although difficult to understand, there is a definite attempt at her name: 'Eywen'. She then gets up and walks, with no difficulty, to a box of toys. She finds a crayon and starts scribbling in circular motions on a red book. You are not sure she should be doing this so you remove the book, at which point she clearly says 'No'. Realising time will be of the essence you ask what colour the book is. She frowns and returns to the table. She starts making a tower of bricks with little difficulty. The examiner asks if there is anything you would like to ask her mother. Mother says she has little difficulty in understanding her but the nursery has raised concerns. She appreciates her speech can be difficult to understand. At this points Helen's five-brick tower crashes to the ground.

How can you assess Helen further?

Where should she be referred?

STATION 7

This station assesses your ability to communicate appropriate, factually correct information in an effective way within the emotional context of the clinical setting:

- **Communication One**

This is a 9-minute station consisting of spoken interaction. You will have up to 2 minutes before the start of the station to read this sheet and prepare yourself. You may make notes on the paper provided.

When the bell sounds you will be invited into the examination room. Please take this instruction sheet with you. The examiner will not ask questions during the 9 minutes but will warn you when you have approximately 2 minutes left.

You are not required to examine a patient.

The encounter should be focused on the task; you will be penalised for asking irrelevant questions or providing superfluous information. You will be marked on your ability to communicate, not the speed with which you convey information. You may not have time to complete the communication.

SETTING

You are the specialist registrar on a general paediatric ward.

SCENARIO

You have reviewed Laura, a 3-year-old who has been admitted for the fifth time this year with acute asthma. You are informed by the GP that no repeat prescriptions have been picked up for Laura in the past 6 months and that Avril, her mother, is a heavy smoker.

TASK

You are meeting with her mother Avril and need to address how she manages her asthma at home and specifically advise her on the risks of smoking.

This station assesses your ability to communicate appropriate, factually correct information in an effective way within the emotional context of the clinical setting:

- Communication Two

This is a 9-minute station consisting of spoken interaction. You will have up to 2 minutes before the start of the station to read this sheet and prepare yourself. You may make notes on the paper provided.

When the bell sounds you will be invited into the examination room. Please take this instruction sheet with you. The examiner will not ask questions during the 9 minutes but will warn you when you have approximately 2 minutes left.

You are not required to examine a patient.

The encounter should be focused on the task; you will be penalised for asking irrelevant questions or providing superfluous information. You will be marked on your ability to communicate, not the speed with which you convey information. You may not have time to complete the communication.

SETTING

You are the specialist registrar on the neonatal unit.

SCENARIO

You are leading a teaching session for the unit's medical students on examination of the newborn. You have been provided with a dislocated hip mannequin.

TASK

Instruct Craig, a fourth-year medical student, on the correct technique for the neonatal hip exam. You do not need to provide background epidemiological information about developmental dysplasia of the hip but if you have time you may check Craig's understanding of what to do if an abnormal hip is discovered. The aim is for Craig to perform a professional, reproducible and effective hip examination on the mannequin in a role-play situation.

STATION 9

This station assesses your ability to take a focused history and explain to the parent your diagnosis or differential management plan:

- **History-taking and Management planning**

This is a 22-minute station of spoken interaction. You will have up to 4 minutes beforehand to prepare yourself. The scenario is below. Be aware you should focus on the task given. You will be penalised for asking irrelevant questions or providing superfluous information. When the bell sounds you will be invited into the examination room. You will have 13 minutes with the patient (with a warning when you have 4 minutes left). You will then have a short period to reflect on the case while the patient leaves the room. You will then have 9 minutes with the examiner.

INFORMATION

You are the SpR in a general paediatric clinic. You receive the following letter from a local orthopaedic consultant. Please take a relevant history from the patient, Tamsin, and her mother:

Dear Colleague,
Re: Tamsin 13 years,

Thank you for seeing Tamsin. She is a 13-year-old girl with a long history of juvenile idiopathic arthritis. I have performed a number of operations on her and most recently an osteotomy of her left hip. This operation was 3 months ago and I understand she is still not back at school. I would be grateful if you could offer your expertise in smoothing her return to education.

Yours sincerely,
Mr A Bone

After taking a history the examiner asks you:

'What is stopping Tamsin going back to school?'

'Who needs to be involved in Tamsin's return to school?'

'How do you think her return could be facilitated?'

COMMENTS ON STATION 1

DIAGNOSIS: PERSISTENT DUCTUS ARTERIOSUS

Every candidate has a fear that they will have little positive (or negative) to say to the examiner because they have been unable to examine the child properly. Even worse, they have examined the child properly and still have nothing to say! There are numerous learning points to remember in this type of station and if you remember a few you should always be able to give a professional answer.

1. APPROACH

As we all know from clinical practice, children of this age can be difficult to examine. They are often clingy and may have stranger anxiety. While examining centres try hard to enrol cooperative children they often get tired or can be unpredictable. It is this random nature that makes children so endearing to paediatricians. You should be comfortable with some distraction techniques for children from 6 months to 5 years. Here are some classics:

Ask mother to show the child a colourful book while you listen to their chest.
Tap a wooden tongue depressor on the desk to attract attention.
Ask the child if you can guess what they had for breakfast by listening to their abdomen (and chest) with your stethoscope.
Does the child have a dummy?
Start listening to teddy's heart, lungs, abdomen, etc., or mother's arm, leg, etc., so the child feels more comfortable.
If you say, 'May I listen to your heart?' and the child says 'No' then you have dug a large hole for yourself. 'I am going to …' should avoid this catastrophe.

Always try to smile and appear unthreatening, despite the stress you are under. Children are unfortunately good at picking up on this. Never carry on regardless if a child becomes very distressed as this will in turn distress the examiner! If a child becomes uncooperative they will often direct you with an alternative plan. Remember there is a tick box in the exam for acknowledging an uncooperative child.

2. OBSERVATION

Before you begin your hands-on exam ask 'mum' to remove any clothing. It will be impossible to pass a station if you miss a scar and you cannot claim you have thoroughly looked unless the chest is exposed.

With a child of this age observation is absolutely vital as it should give you enough information to make a sensible list of possible diagnoses. In the above scenario we need to simply stand back and take a look for a minute.

We note that she sits without oxygen and is not cyanosed or dyspnoeic.

- If she has a cardiac defect it is acyanotic.

We look more carefully and notice she is small for her age, has plagiocephaly and on inspection of the dorsum of her hands has multiple scars, presumably from previous venepuncture.

- She has signs of being premature.

As mum distracts her and removes her T-shirt you carefully inspect her chest and both axillae. Now you can see a healed left lateral thoracotomy incision. She has had surgery for either:

- aortic coarctation repair;
- pulmonary artery (PA) banding;
- a Blalock–Taussig (BT) shunt;
- persistent ductus arteriosus (PDA); or
- surgery on the left lung itself.

In the absence of a central sternotomy scar she has not had a BT shunt as she is pink. Remember, a BT shunt is a palliative procedure and will not reverse the cause of the cyanosis. PA banding is used to prepare the vessels for a Fontan procedure but again will not correct the cyanosis until a more definitive repair has been performed. This leaves (given that this is a cardiac station) only a PDA or coarctation repair as possibilities. We know her pulses are normal, although if the coarctation has been repaired then obviously you will be able to feel the femoral pulse. In this situation, if a classical repair has been used then the left radial pulse should be weak. Balloon dilatation of the coarctation is unlikely to show any discernible difference. So theoretically the child may have had an aortic coarctation or a PDA but we know she shows signs of being premature. Therefore, if Hannah became very distressed and uncooperative you would be able to say to the examiner:

'Hannah is a 12-month-old girl. She is not attached to any monitoring or supplementary oxygen. On inspection she is pink in air with no respiratory distress. I note she has plagiocephaly and her hands show scars consistent with multiple venepuncture. She appears small for her age but I would like to plot her on a growth chart. On examination of the precordium Hannah has a left lateral thoracotomy scar. I was unable to proceed further with my examination but this acyanotic child has features of prematurity and a left lateral thoracotomy scar which would make a repaired persistent ductus arteriosus the most likely diagnosis.'

In this way you should be able to pass the station without ever having heard a heart sound! Obviously this system is not so helpful if the primary lesion is a ventriculoseptal defect! But to give yourself at least a sporting chance it is vital you use all the clues you are given.

REMINDERS

Remember your caveat for the end of the cardiovascular examination?

'I would like to complete my examination by taking a blood pressure, oxygen saturation level and plotting him/her on a growth chart appropriate for age and sex.'

CAN YOU …

Describe two common features of persistent ductus arteriosus? See page 164.

COMMENTS ON STATION 2

DIAGNOSIS: KIDNEY TRANSPLANT

Obviously it is vital to palpate the mass in this station, and only regular practice of feeling abdomens (easily overlooked in favour of the more classic chest exam) will help you do this. However, you need to know what the mass is to make sense of the station. The common pelvic masses – and note pelvic, not abdominal – are:

1. Palpable bladder
2. Inflammatory mass – unlikely if well and non-tender
3. Constipation
4. Renal transplant
5. Ovarian pathology (must be a girl!).

Simon has signs of a chronic disease (pallor, suboptimal growth, multiple surgery). This situation would fit very well with chronic renal disease and a kidney transplant. Simon had developed chronic renal failure secondary due to vesicoureteric reflux complicated by persistent and undertreated/missed urinary tract infection. He required peritoneal dialysis (hence two hypochondrial scars) and a short period of haemodialysis (hence the healed central line scar close to the clavicle) and was later successfully transplanted with a donor kidney. Easy when you know! You wouldn't be able to tell the cause of the chronic renal failure in this case but must know the common causes and any potential features to look for.

It is useful to commit a list of investigations to memory as some are specific for renal problems and just saying, 'FBC, U&Es, CRP' etc. is unlikely to win you any favours.

- Monitoring
  - Blood pressure
  - Urinalysis
- Iron studies
  - Full blood count *and* ferritin
- Renal function
  - Urea and electrolytes
  - Creatinine
  - Bicarbonate
  - Measurement of GFR (radioisotope scan)

Causes of chronic renal failure

Disease	Cause	Features
Renal scarring	Multiple UTIs Vesicoureteric reflux	Has the child got spina bifida?
Glomerulonephritis	Henoch–Schönlein purpura Vasculitides	Any joint swelling or arthralgia? Purpura?
Hereditary	Polycystic kidney disease Cystinosis Alport's syndrome	Are the parents well? Hearing difficulty?
Congenital dysplasia		
Systemic	Tumours SLE	Butterfly rash

- Nutritional status
  - Albumin
  - Protein
- Renal osteodystrophy
  - Calcium
  - Phosphate
  - Alkaline phosphatase
  - Left wrist X-ray
- Renal imaging
  - Ultrasound

Complications of chronic renal failure (or more relevantly features to look for and so avoid deterioration) are split between those of the disease or those of the surgical treatment (i.e., transplant).

Prior to the exam make sure you get to see a few children with renal problems as they are not uncommon in the exam. Be familiar with the appearance and location of peritoneal dialysis catheters and central lines used for haemodialysis. Renal nurses are a mine of useful information in this regard.

Remember, there is a significant psychosocial burden and counselling, family therapy and social service input may have to be sought.

At the end of your abdominal exam remember your caveat: 'I would like to complete my examination by performing a blood pressure, urinalysis and plotting on a growth chart appropriate for age and sex'.

CAN YOU …

List the investigations you would perform in a child you suspect has chronic renal failure?

Pre-treatment	Treatment	Post-treatment
Hypertension	Control medically: Beta-blocker (care asthma) Furosemide (care potassium) Must involve nephrologists	Dialysis – complications Peritonitis Volume depletion Dialysate leakage Transplant – complications Infection – particularly CMV Must prevent UTI Rejection Immunosuppression
Metabolic acidosis	Sodium citrate solutions (care: sodium may worsen hypertension)	
Growth failure	Growth hormone	
Renal osteodystrophy	Dietary phosphate restriction Phosphate binders Vitamin D	
Uraemic symptoms (anorexia, nausea and lethargy)	Dietary protein restriction	
Anaemia	Erythropoietin	
Seizures (hypertensive or electrolyte imbalance)		
If poor concentrating power: Polyuria Salt wasting		

REMINDER

Renal osteodystrophy

1. Poorly functioning kidneys unable to convert (hydroxylate) vitamin D to its active form.
2. Vitamin D needed to absorb calcium (mainly intestinal dietary calcium).
3. Calcium subsequently falls.
4. Parathyroid hormone (PTH) increases to compensate by increasing bone resorption of calcium.
5. Without treatment calcium levels stay low. Increasing PTH causes further excessive bone demineralisation.
6. As kidney function falls, the excretion of phosphate (aided by PTH) becomes inadequate.
7. This further increases PTH (with no effect on phosphate excretion due to the kidney's poor function), thereby increasing bone demineralisation.
8. Treatment: phosphate restriction by diet and binding with calcium carbonate; increase calcium by giving vitamin D supplements.

Renal transplants

Renal transplants may be from live donors or cadaveric. They are usually located in the pelvis with the native kidneys left in. Occasionally the native kidneys are removed prior to transplantation, so remember to look at the sides and back for scars too. You may sometimes see a scar or plaster from a renal biopsy to give you a clue.

Abdominal masses

Palpating an abdominal mass which isn't a liver or spleen is not common in your average paediatric take. Although you may have learnt a great deal about paediatric gastrointestinal conditions it is useful having a list of the paediatric causes of abdominal masses. Running through these with the examiner and explaining how they fit the clinical picture presented will buy you time if you really are stumped as to the cause of an odd lump.

The table below does not include medical causes of hepatosplenomegaly as this is a list in its own right. Apart from gastrointestinal causes you will see that it is very unlikely any of the following will appear in the exam. Therefore think very carefully about offering them as a diagnosis.

Causes of abdominal mass in children (not including hepatosplenomegaly)

Gastrointestinal	Liver	Genitourinary	Other
Inflammatory mass: • Crohn's • Post-appendectomy Constipation Pyloric stenosis	Choledochal cyst Hepatoblastoma	Renal mass: • Hydronephrosis • Nephroblastoma • Urethral valves	Neuroblastoma Sarcoma

COMMENTS ON STATION 3

DIAGNOSIS: PREVIOUS MASTOIDECTOMY

Abdi is an 11-year-old Somalian boy with a left-sided facial weakness affecting all the muscles on that side. The sensation to his face appears normal. Tuning fork tests reveal a left-sided conductive hearing problem. I must look at his left auditory meatus and drum but I suspect there may be some signs of chronic damage. Abdi may have had a mastoidectomy performed, as evidenced by the scarring behind his left ear. It may be this child has had chronic otitis media and mastoiditis. The seventh nerve palsy which is of the lower motor neurone may have been a result of the original infection or of the surgical treatment.

Severe, untreated otitis media may present with a facial nerve palsy. It is uncommon in the United Kingdom (but not unheard of) due to the use of antibiotics. In fact there is a feeling in some countries that mastoiditis is on the increase as GPs use antibiotics less for otitis media.

Although we rarely use tuning forks in clinical practice it is one of those things that occasionally comes up in the exam and can flummox candidates if you don't refresh your memory. Tuning fork tests are based on the principle that sound should travel better through air than through bone in the absence of hearing impairment. Weber's test is performed by placing a vibrating 512 Hz tuning fork on the vertex of the skull. If the patient, when asked, can hear the sound louder on one side compared to the other then this is abnormal. The side the sound is localised to indicates conductive hearing loss on that side or sensory hearing loss on the contralateral side. Rinne's test involves placing a vibrating fork next to the pinna (testing air conduction) and then behind the pinna on the mastoid process (testing bone conduction). If the sound is heard better through air than through bone then it is said to be Rinne's positive and vice versa. Rinne's test is positive in sensorineural hearing loss or normal hearing and negative in conductive hearing loss.

In this case:

- Weber's lateralises to the left
- Rinne's positive on the right
- Rinne's negative on the left.

One word of warning – and ignore this if you think it will confuse you: with the above findings it is still possible that there is a sensorineural or perceptive defect on the right side. This is because Rinne's may be positive on the right because of a sensorineural deficit (and not due to normal hearing). The Weber's lateralises to the left because there is some bone conduction on the left side. It would be unlucky to have had mastoiditis on the left side and have a sensorineural deafness on the right. You should be aware of this if asked, although it is probably best not to volunteer that information.

It is important to be able to quickly examine different cranial nerves. You are unlikely to be expected to perform an examination of all the nerves due to time constraints. Practise, practise, practise, as being slick under pressure is important and the cranial nerve exam is easy to perform on housemates.

Bell's palsy is an easy condition to bring to the exam. There is some variation in textbooks as to recovery but as a general rule:

- 80–90% will make a full recovery in 3–6 months.
- The remainder have a mild residual weakness of the nerve.
- A small proportion (up to 5%) will have a permanent and unfortunately severe nerve deficit.

You must remember that methylcellulose eye-drops (artificial tears) need to be prescribed and the eye may need to be taped at night. The use of steroids depends on local guidelines but a short 2 mg/kg course is often recommended.

REMINDER

Physiologically, but not practically, examination of the seventh nerve is completed by testing taste in the anterior two-thirds of the mouth.

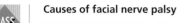
Causes of facial nerve palsy

Upper motor neurone lesion		Lower motor neurone lesion	
Intracranial tumour	Any behaviour change? Vomiting? Signs of raised ICP?	Bell's palsy	Only diagnosed if the below are excluded
Cerebral palsy	Characteristic peripheral motor signs	Ramsay Hunt	Check for vesicles in the auditory canal
Möbius' syndrome	Congenital facial diplegia (absence of the nerve nuclei)	Chronic otitis media	Examine eardrum
		Hypertension	Blood pressure
		Intracranial tumour	Any behaviour change? Vomiting? Signs of raised ICP?
		Infections	EBV Mumps Lyme disease Guillain–Barré (but usually bilateral)
		Skull fracture/injury	Birth history (?forceps)
		Leukaemia	Rare but may be first presenting symptom

CAN YOU …

Talk through your history and examination of the child you suspect may have a Bell's palsy?

COMMENTS ON STATION 4

DIAGNOSIS: ATOPIC ECZEMA

The moral of this story is: stick to your guns! The patient in this case does have atopic eczema and mild asthma. He is currently well, however, and has no clinical signs of asthma. *Never* make up clinical signs as it will land you in a whole heap of trouble. The examiners want to see safe, reliable doctors and not imaginative ones! They need to be confident that when phoned at 3 o'clock in the morning you have not made up signs to fit a given clinical picture. If you think you may have difficulty saying there are no clinical signs when you think there should be, then you can always acknowledge this:

'Anthony is a well-grown 6-year-old with eczema. Eczema is associated with other atopic conditions such as asthma and hay fever. He has no wheeze or

signs of chronic respiratory distress on examination at present. However, it would be important to take a good history from Anthony and his parents to ensure he has no interval symptoms.'

Each centre will have a variety of patients with a variety of clinical signs. Not all of them will be obvious or even present at the time of the exam. Be prepared for this. Also, make sure that you read the question. In the above question you were asked to listen to the chest (as opposed to examining the respiratory system). Don't waste the examiner's time or your own by starting at the hands. The examiner will probably have other tasks he wants you to perform.

You should have a sound understanding of the management of basic paediatric problems that you are likely to see in clinic as an SpR, such as eczema and asthma.

Ezcema

Diagnosis	May present in infancy onwards Family or personal history of atopy
Management: non-medical	Switch to a non-biological washing powder Trim fingernails Use mittens in the persistent child
Management: medical	*Emollient*: Apply generously. Examples include 50:50 paraffin. Avoid soap and use bath oils such as Oilatum. Some bath oils include antiseptic, such as Emulsiderm *Steroid cream:* Use sparingly on troublesome areas. Be wary of using too high a strength. 0.5–1% hydrocortisone on the face or on babies. Stronger steroid creams include: • *Eumovate*: Moderately potent • *Betnovate*: Potent • *Dermovate*: Very potent Creams can be used on the body of older children if only for short periods of time. The flexures are prone to atrophy with prolonged treatment. Oral steroid (prednisolone) has a role in difficult or acute eczema *Topical tacrolimus ointment*: A newer treatment. 0.03% cream may be suitable in children where topical steroid has not worked or they are at particular risk of steroid skin atrophy. Normally initiated by a dermatologist *Wet wraps*: Potassium permanganate soaks may be used or ichthammol bandages over steroid and emollient held in place by Tubigrip. These are changed every 1–3 days *Antimicrobials*: Systemic antibiotics generally preferred if indicated. Intravenous antibiotics are sometimes indicated in more severe cases of infected eczema. Herpetic eczema is an emergency requiring treatment with acyclovir *Immunosuppressants*: These may be required in severe refractory eczema under the guidance of a dermatologist. Ciclosporin and azathioprine are the more commonly used drugs of choice

COMMENTS ON STATION 5

DIAGNOSIS: WILLIAMS' SYNDROME

This question is another example of the need to be versatile. You may be asked to perform small, separate tasks. In this question it is important to be able to interact well with a child and think on your feet. Don't be thrown by simple questions such as 'Look at this. What do you think?' – a difficult skill to revise for but may be practised by asking friends to pretend to be syndromes and feed you snippets of their features until you recognise them. You may not be able to spot the particular feature in the exam but you will start to learn certain patterns of abnormality.

We learn quite quickly from Nicola that she has some intellectual impairment and soft dysmorphic features, so any number of general questions may be appropriate.

Does Nicola attend a mainstream school?
Does Nicola have a statement of special educational needs/special educational needs coordinator?
Is Nicola under the care of a community paediatrician?
Did Nicola spend time in SCBU/NICU?
Is she growing well?

We then see that Nicola has evidence of previous cardiac surgery with no residual murmurs. It is impossible to say what surgery she has had, although the absence of thoracotomy scars indicates that a shunting procedure was unnecessary.

So … dysmorphic features; intellectual impairment; cardiac problems. There are a few syndromes that may have this collection of difficulties:

- Down's
- Di George's
- Noonan's
- Williams'
- Alagille's
- Fetal alcohol.

(Tuberous sclerosis and neurofibromatosis do *not* have cardiac defects as part of their clinical and associated features.)

The other clue we have above is her very happy, chatty demeanour. This is characteristic of Williams' syndrome (and Down's but the phenotypic features are not present). In the case of Williams' the textbooks would describe it as 'cocktail party chatter' but do not expect this to be obviously apparent. There is no substitution for actually having seen the condition described as opposed to having simply read about it.

With this in mind you could ask mum and the examiner some clever questions to show that you know what you're talking about.

Did Nicola have problems with high calcium levels as a baby?

Did she have an operation due to supravalvular aortic stenosis?

Is Nicola gifted at music?

Or if you're feeling really clever: has she had FISH studies to show she has a problem with chromosome 7?

REMINDER

Williams' syndrome

Facial	Systemic	Clinical
Prominent lips	Hypoplastic nails	Transient neonatal
Blue eyes	Supravalvular aortic stenosis	hypercalcaemia
Microdontia	Pulmonary artery stenosis	Mild IUGR
Snub nose	Renal artery stenosis	Mild microcephaly
Medial eyebrow flare		Mild learning difficulties
Stellate pattern to iris		
Short palpebral fissures		

COMMENTS ON STATION 6

DIAGNOSIS: ISOLATED SPEECH DELAY/SPEECH DIFFICULTY

As is emphasised repeatedly in the book, it is vital to have a fluid understanding of key developmental stages. You should be able to pick out the following features:

- Gross motor
  - Walks well: at least 18 months
- Fine motor
  - Circular scribble: at least 18 months
  - Tower of five bricks: 18–24 months
- Speech/hearing
  - At least three words: at least 12–15 months
  - Communicates wishes: at least 12–15 months
- Social
  - Plays independently: around 18 months.

Although the station implied delayed speech and language, the question demanded a complete developmental age assessment. Without doing any formal assessment the above has already given you a good framework in which to calculate any potential delays. In this brief segment you see a child who is probably 18–24 months with a potential speech and hearing delay. However, it is likely the child has a good vocabulary and the problem is with articulation. You can test this by asking her to point to and then say the name of well-recognisable objects.

When listening to speech it is important to appreciate the difference between:

- Mechanical problems:
  - *Dysarthria*: a weakness of the muscles used for speaking or dysfunction of the neural pathways used to coordinate speech, resulting in difficulty in forming and speaking words.
  - *Dysphonia*: an abnormality to the sound or phonation of speech. This implies damage to the recurrent laryngeal nerve (tenth cranial nerve).
- Developmental problems: this encompasses a delay due to familial, environmental or central causes.

It is important to exclude factors such as poor input at home. This would suggest emotional deprivation or simply that parents do not or are unable to speak to their child regularly at home. Bear in mind autism, cerebral palsy or generalised developmental delay.

It is also important to remember that language problems may be receptive or expressive. Receptive language develops earlier and may begin to become appreciable from the age of 9 months. By the first year of life the child may understand 20–50 words. There is a sudden acceleration in both components from approximately 18 months. An expressive disorder may be present when the child's vocabulary is actually quite good. A child may be able to point to multiple named objects but not able to say them.

It is difficult to know if Helen's speech problems are part of a normal spectrum of delayed adequate phonation or represent a specific mechanical problem. In the absence of other features of developmental delay it would be most appropriate to refer this child to a speech and language therapist or health visitor. It may be that a speech and language therapist will delay active therapy until the child is older, however.

CAN YOU …

Examine the ninth, tenth, eleventh and twelfth cranial nerves?
(Look away now and talk through your examination with a colleague or in the mirror. Don't cheat!)

- *Ninth*: glossopharyngeal nerve
  - *Motor*: stylopharyngeal muscle (raises the pharynx). However, the palatopharyngeal muscle (CN X) also performs this action so difficult to assess in isolation.
  - *Sensory*: supplies the posterior third of the tongue (but not likely to be performed in the exam!)
- *Tenth*: vagus nerve
  - *Motor*: nerves to pharynx and larynx. Tested by gag and palatal reflex. Neither will endear you to the examiner or child if

performed. However, the palatal reflex (touching the soft palate causes it to lift) may be performed if specifically requested.

- *Eleventh*: spinal accessory nerve
  - *Motor*: Shrug shoulders (trapezius). Push jaw into hand placed on the medial side of the face with the head turned to one side (sternocleidomastoid).
- *Twelfth*: hypoglossal
  - *Motor*: Check for fasciculation of the tongue first (easily forgotten). This is a sign of lower motor neurone lesion. Ask the child to stick out their tongue, which deviates to the side of the lesion.

A thorough working knowledge of cranial nerve exam is assumed but the above has been included as revision tends to concentrate on the earlier nerves!

COMMENTS ON STATION 7

The key to success in the communication skills is not only having the required communication skills to impress the examiner with your empathy, non-lexical utterances and engagement but also to provide the information the question asks for. In this scenario you are going to have to spend some time obtaining background on the mother's understanding of her child's condition (why is she not picking up repeat prescriptions?), explaining the need for regular medication and then giving generic advice on smoking. It is vital you do not get too involved in Laura's current state of health and how Laura is being managed at the moment. The role-player will not drag you down this route but will not stop you if you do!

The station is underpinned by how Laura's mother understands asthma. Has she been poorly informed on previous admissions and is not using medication correctly? Or is there an element of neglect in her care of her child? It is unlikely you will be given a child protection issue to investigate, although you must acknowledge to the examiner by your questions that you may be concerned by this:

Are any other health professionals (health visitor, for instance) involved in her care?
Does she have other children to look after?
How does she feel she is coping with Laura's asthma?

The role-player will have been given background on her character (which you will not be party to) and will have an individual interpretation on this. Examples may be:

You are: The mother of one child, Laura, who was diagnosed with asthma a year ago.
Background information: You are a busy single working mother who is struggling with working and raising a child at the same time. Laura is repeatedly unwell and has required multiple hospital admissions. On each occasion you have found the doctors too busy to take a little extra time to explain Laura's treatment plan with you. You did not want to

impose on them and were grateful to leave the hospital quickly so you could get back to work. The inhalers you have been given seem still to be working, so you have never felt the need to pick up further prescriptions.

Your general feelings:

- You have been increasingly worried about Laura's health recently and feel maybe it is time to get to grips with the situation. You would also like to stop smoking but don't know how to get the support.

After the doctor has explained the situation to you, your feelings and possible further questions may be:

- How do I get advice on the correct way to give Laura her medication?
- Don't steroids impair growth?
- It's very difficult to stop smoking. Is there anyone who can help?
- Will Laura always be like this?

Compare the above story with the following:

You are: The mother of five children. Laura, the middle of the five, was diagnosed with asthma a year ago.

Background information: Three of your children have or have had asthma, of whom Laura is the youngest. Your oldest child, now twelve, appears to have grown out of his asthma. The second oldest, 7 years old, is very rarely ill although it appears your 1½-year-old is developing symptoms. You also have a 2-month-old child.

   You are confident in dealing with asthma but do not acknowledge that Laura appears to have been into hospital much more frequently than her siblings. You have been using her older brother's inhaler to avoid having to go to the GP.

   Both yourself and your partner are heavy smokers but never smoke in the same room as your children. Your mother smoked when you were younger and you don't appear to have come to any harm.

Your general feelings:

- You are not unduly concerned by Laura's health as you feel she will eventually get better.

After the doctor has explained the situation to you, your feelings and possible further questions may be:

- If she will get better anyway why do I have to give her the steroids? They are bad, aren't they?
- I don't smoke in the same room as the children, so why should I give up?
- It's difficult to organise trips to the GP/hospital so I don't want to come to any follow-up.

Obviously these are very different scenarios, although the information presented to you is the same. Being open to or trying to predict the background information will help you form a framework for the station. In this situation it is obviously vital to discover how many children the mother has, but you may not necessarily think to ask that question.

   It will be useful to practise making up scenarios with colleagues (who are preferably taking the exam).

REMINDER

You may remember the term 'non-lexical utterances' from communication skills at medical school. These are small noises or prompts, which are not true words, that act as an encouragement to the person you are speaking to. They are often associated with nodding motions of the head or arm gestures. Examples include 'Mmmmm', 'Ahhhh', 'Uh-huh'. Some candidates will use them almost subconsciously.

COMMENTS ON STATION 8

The communication station is always underpinned by having a thorough knowledge of the subject being discussed. It is assumed that the candidate knows the required technique, base knowledge or has the requested information to answer the child's or parent's question. If candidates display to the examiner a lack of understanding of the basic principles required of a specialist registrar, it will be difficult to justify a pass regardless of the strength of their communication skills. This station requires that you actually know how to explain the science behind the hip exam, not just simply push the hips open and closed. The emphasis will be on your ability to communicate an apparently simple procedure, albeit with a complex mechanism, in a concise and informative manner.

1. Introduce yourself. Ask the student's name and understanding of the topic.
2. Explain the objectives of the session:
   - To introduce the concept of the neonatal hip examination.
   - What abnormal features you may find on inspection.
   - You must explain your examination procedure to the parents so they do not become distressed at your actions.
   - Discussion of Barlow's and Ortolani's tests.
   - Practical demonstration.
   - Ensure correct student procedure.
   - Ask if the student has any questions.
3. Neonatal hip examination is a screening procedure carried out on every child born in the UK. The screening is for developmental dysplasia of the hip (DDH); avoid the term 'congenital dislocation'. There is a repeat test by the GP at 6 weeks of age.
4. DDH may present with asymmetrical skin creases or an apparent shortening of the femur (Galeazzi's sign). These features are unlikely to present at birth and are more likely to be apparent at the 6-week check.
5. You must inform the parents that you will be opening and closing the hips. This will not hurt the child but they may not like the sensation and so may become upset.
6. *Barlow's test*: The child must be lying on their back with the hips flexed at approximately 90° to the abdomen and heels touching the buttocks. Keeping the knee fully flexed, place your thumb on the medial condyle of the femur. Your fingers should be placed on the greater trochanter so that you have complete control of the femur and will not be touching the hip. These landmarks may be difficult to find in the chunky neonate. It is most important that the student is seen to have a good grip on the femur

and has their thumb on the medial aspect and fingers on the lateral aspect of the thigh. Pushing down on the hip following a line of force through the femur may demonstrate the 'clunk' of hip dislocation – a positive Barlow's test.

7. *Ortolani's test*: This test relocates a dislocated hip. With hands in the same position as in Barlow's test, you must simultaneously abduct (open out) the hips and provide an anterior force on the femur (i.e., the opposite to Barlow's test). This may produce the 'clunk' of reduction – a positive Ortolani test.

8. In practice, both hips are examined at the same time and both Barlow's and Ortolani's tests are performed in one 'in and out' motion. For the purposes of student demonstration it may be best to focus on one hip and one procedure.

9. The hip dummy tends to have one hip which obviously comes out of place. If this is the case the student must demonstrate his ability to produce and recognise hip dislocation. You will fail the station if there is the possibility the student may not be able to correctly identify DDH. You will not fail the station if you run out of time.

10. Ask the student to demonstrate their understanding by asking them to role-play an exam with you as parent of the hip dummy. He must introduce himself, explain the procedure and perform the test. If you have time you can then discuss what he would say to parents if the test is positive.

REMINDER

DDH

Epidemiology

- Girls > boys
- Left > right
- Risk factors:
  - Breech
  - Family history (first degree – not a second cousin once removed!)
  - Talipes calcaneovalgus
  - Oligohydramnios
- Neuromuscular disorders.

Screening

- Check your local policy. Those children with risk factors must have an ultrasound regardless of examination findings, although actual criteria differ between units. Universal ultrasound screening is a controversial area and further studies are ongoing as to its effectiveness.

Treatment

- Children with an obvious dislocation at the newborn exam may be referred to the orthopaedic surgeons and splinting commenced as soon as possible. The hip is maintained in flexion and abduction.

Double/triple diapers are frowned upon by some groups but some textbooks still advocate their use.

Unfortunately, some children are missed by screening (potentially the group where the hip acetabulum fails to form as the child grows). Treatment is possible in this group but if the child has begun to walk the painless limp and Trendelenburg gait may be irreversible.

COMMENTS ON STATION 9

Taking a history in itself is a simple task by now and something we all do on a day-to-day basis. The key to this station is asking the relevant questions pertinent to the scenario. In this situation the examiner would certainly forgive you for not asking about immunisations and allergies but would expect a detailed probe into her disabilities. Time in this station is pressured. Pressure contributes to mistakes. Mistakes contribute to failing.

The following is a review of Tamsin's history. Assume that Tamsin and her mother would not have revealed information without a direct question about that information. Write down the questions you would have asked Tamsin. How much of the following information would you have gleaned?

Tamsin has had severe juvenile chronic arthritis since 4 years of age and has tried many different drug therapies. She has many affected joints and associated impairments. She requires help from her mother with dressing, toileting and bathing. She is able to walk but requires a wheelchair for longer distances. She has missed many months of schooling over the years. Tamsin and her mother receive no help at home and Tamsin's mother is a full-time carer but is only claiming unemployment benefit. Her mother has a car but it doesn't fit a wheelchair. Nothing has been put in place to help Tamsin at school.

None of the above is really 'medical'. Obtaining the above information is vital as without it you will not pass the station. Of course, it is important to classify the type of arthritis, previous and current treatment, presence of antibodies, etc., but the child's functional ability will be of more interest to the examiner. Remember you are not the on-call SHO but the clinic-based registrar for this station.

There are many reasons why Tamsin may find it difficult to go back to school.

Emotionally:

- She is bullied for being 'short'.
- She only has one friend due to the time she has missed.
- She is self-conscious about her joint deformities.
- She struggles due to the work that is missed.

Physically:

- She needs help with toileting and dressing at school.
- She is unable to take flights of stairs to different lessons.
- She needs transport to and from school.

To enable Tamsin's return to school many people need to be involved:

Tamsin
Tamsin's parents
GP
School nurse
Head teacher
Community physiotherapist
Occupational therapist
Social services
?Community paediatrician.

By getting all these people together plans can be put into place to enable Tamsin to return to school. This is what the examiner will be looking for.

REMINDER

The juvenile arthritides are an easily confusing group of conditions.

Name	Frequency	Onset	Test	Eye involvement (uveitis)
Systemic	10–20%	Early childhood	RF and ANA negative	Nil
Oligoarticular (persistent) < 4 joints	40–50%	2–5 years	ANA positivity increases risk of uveitis	Yes (need regular slit lamp exam)
Oligoarticular (extended) > 5 joints after 6 months	5–10%	2–5 years	RF negative	Yes
Polyarticular (rheumatoid factor negative)	15–20%	Childhood	RF negative ANA positive 25%	Rare
Polyarticular (rheumatoid factor positive)	5–10%	Late childhood	RF positive ANA positive 50–70%	Rare
Psoriatic	8–10%	Throughout childhood	RF negative ANA positive 20–50%	Potential

RF, rheumatoid factor; ANA, antinuclear antibody negative.

Circuit B

STATION 1

This station assesses your ability to elicit clinical signs:

- **CVS**

This is a 9-minute station of clinical interaction. You will have up to 4 minutes beforehand to prepare yourself. No additional information will be given or is necessary before commencing the station. When the bell sounds you will be invited into the examination room.

INTRODUCTION

The examiner tells you, 'This patient has recently changed practice areas and the GP is concerned about this 4-month-old child's growth. Can you examine this child's cardiovascular system to determine a cause for his poor weight gain?'.

CLINICAL SCENARIO

You are presented with a child who looks small for his age. He obviously has Down's syndrome.

What cardiac defects would you predict this child may have?

The child is placid throughout the examination. On general inspection his lips are not cyanosed and you note dysmorphology consistent with Down's syndrome. Examination of peripheral pulses reveals no delay or absence in any area. The pulse is 120–130.

On examination of the sternum you can see an obvious cardiac impulse. The apex can be felt just medial to the axillary line at the level of the fourth intercostal space. Both first and second heart sounds are present, although you suspect the second heart sound is louder than the first. There is a loud murmur without a thrill heard at the lower left sternal border. The chest is clear and a liver edge is just palpable below the left subcostal margin.

What do you say to the examiner?

STATION 2

This station assesses your ability to elicit clinical signs:
- **Abdo/Other**

INTRODUCTION

The examiner asks, 'Can you introduce yourself to Sarah and make some general comments about her appearance?'.

CLINICAL SCENARIO

Sarah is a small preschool-appearing child who is able to say hello to you and tell you her name. She tells you she is 6 years old. You say to the examiner you would like to plot her height and weight on a growth chart as she appears small for age. You note a relatively large abdomen with some peripheral muscle wasting. You comment that she does not appear dysmorphic.

The examiner asks you to complete a full abdominal examination.

After a thorough examination of her hands, skin and eyes you can find no palmar erythema, clubbing, jaundice or spider naevi but do note some haematological dysfunction in the fact she has multiple bruises. These are not solely located on the shins but encompass the arms and thighs as well. They are of multiple colours and shades.

Her abdomen is protuberant but soft and non-tender. You feel an obviously enlarged liver (at least the width of your hand) but after a thorough exam cannot feel the spleen. You are surprised to find you are able to feel potential renal masses on both flanks. The liver is not tender to palpate.

Are there any other physical signs you wish to specifically wish to look at?

Are there any questions you wish to ask Sarah's mother?

Is there a diagnosis which brings all these features together?

STATION 3

This station assesses your ability to elicit clinical signs:
- **Neurological**

This is a 9-minute station of clinical interaction. You will have up to 4 minutes beforehand to prepare yourself. No additional information will be given or is necessary before commencing the station. When the bell sounds you will be invited into the examination room.

INTRODUCTION

On entering the room the examiner says to you, 'Please examine the back of this 6-month-old boy and then proceed to examine where else you feel necessary'.

CLINICAL SCENARIO

You are presented with a young infant who is lying on his back on an examining table. You introduce yourself to his mother and gain permission to examine the child's back. Quickly, but obviously, you scan the child before turning him over. There is no obvious dysmorphism, the child is not grossly hypotonic and the hips are flexed. He is only wearing a nappy and smiles as you approach.

On turning him over there is an obvious large scar in the lumbosacral region. It is in the midline and looks at least a couple of months old.

Which areas of the body could you justify examining now?

You elect to examine the lower limbs. On close inspection he does not appear grossly wasted. There are no fasciculations and there is some intermittent kicking movement at the knee, although it doesn't appear as coordinated as you would expect in a 6-month-old child. The hips are in a permanent flexed and abducted position. There is no hip extension. The knee is observed to extend but the foot is held in a position of dorsiflexion. You are unable to obtain ankle reflexes but feel happy you have obtained an adequate knee reflex. Babinski's reflex is unequivocal but the child shows no facial response to the test. As you begin to test sensation the examiner asks you to present your findings so far.

This station assesses your ability to elicit clinical signs:
- **Respiratory/Other**

This is a 9-minute station of clinical interaction. You will have up to 4 minutes beforehand to prepare yourself. No additional information will be given or is necessary before commencing the station. When the bell sounds you will be invited into the examination room.

INTRODUCTION

On entering the room you are asked to examine Samantha's respiratory system.

CLINICAL SCENARIO

You are presented with a teenage girl in her late teens who appears exceptionally tall (and too long for the couch!). She is comfortable at rest. On inspection of her hands, she has very long fingers. There is no central cyanosis.

On examination of her chest, she has an increased anteroposterior diameter and marked scoliosis. There is equal expansion but loss of the cardiac dullness on percussion. There are coarse inspiratory crackles at both bases and occasional wheeze. There is no hepatomegaly.

What specific clinical signs will you look for?

STATION 5

This station assesses your ability to elicit clinical signs:

- **Other**

This is a 9-minute station of clinical interaction. You will have up to 4 minutes beforehand to prepare yourself. No additional information will be given or is necessary before commencing the station. When the bell sounds you will be invited into the examination room.

INTRODUCTION

'Please have a close look at Sarah's face and neck. Her GP has noticed a subtle decrease in her height velocity.'

CLINICAL SCENARIO

You are presented with a girl who is approximately 5–7 years old. She has no overt dysmorphology. She engages with you and is able to answer questions about her age – 'Seven' – and where she goes to school. She has a normal voice. You comment to the examiner that you think she has a midline neck swelling.

How would you approach the examination of the neck?

Your examination reveals a diffusely enlarged firm thyroid swelling.

How would you confirm the swelling is an enlarged thyroid?

What other features on systemic exam will you now look for?

STATION 6

This station assesses your ability to assess specifically requested areas in a child with a developmental problem:

- **Development**

This is a 9-minute station of clinical interaction. You will have up to 4 minutes beforehand to prepare yourself. No additional information will be given or is necessary before commencing the station. When the bell sounds you will be invited into the examination room.

INTRODUCTION

On walking into the room you are asked to assess the general development of Katie, who is 1 year old.

CLINICAL SCENARIO

Katie is sitting up in the middle of the room. She has been given a rattle to hold, which she bangs against the ground. She looks up at your approach and drops her rattle. You introduce yourself to her mother and gain permission to examine her. She picks up her rattle, which has fallen behind her. You commence your examination.

Gross motor: Although able to sit up without support, she is unable to stand. With her hands held there is an effort to pull up but she doesn't yet have the strength in her legs. She will roll from front to back or back to front. Her general tone is good and there is no evidence of spasticity.

Fine motor: If she drops her rattle she is able to pick it up (in either hand) with a palmar grasp.

Hearing/language: She responds to her mother's voice by looking at her. You are not given time to do a formal distraction test. She makes noises but no distinguishable words.

Social: She smiles and shows little fear of you. When given a spoon she accidentally hits herself over the head with it.

General: She appears small for her age, and has the composition of an approximately 6-month-old child. There are no dysmorphic features but she does have a plagiocephalic skull and scars on her hands.

What do you say to the examiner?

Why might this child have developmental delay?

STATION 7

This station assesses your ability to communicate appropriate, factually correct information in an effective way within the emotional context of the clinical setting:

- **Communication One**

This is a 9-minute station consisting of spoken interaction. You will have up to 2 minutes before the start of the station to read this sheet and prepare yourself. You may make notes on the paper provided.

When the bell sounds you will be invited into the examination room. Please take this instruction sheet with you. The examiner will not ask questions during the 9 minutes but will warn you when you have approximately 2 minutes left.

You are not required to examine a patient.

The encounter should be focused on the task; you will be penalised for asking irrelevant questions or providing superfluous information. You will be marked on your ability to communicate, not the speed with which you convey information. You may not have time to complete the communication.

SETTING

You are a paediatric registrar in a district general hospital.

SCENARIO

You will be talking to Mrs White, the mother of Hayley, a 3-week-old baby who has been found on Guthrie neonatal screening to have raised immune reactive trypsin and to be likely to have CF. She has been asked to come to the hospital for the results and further management to be explained.

TASK

Explain the results of the Guthrie test to Mrs White and the necessary next steps in management. You must sensitively respond to all of Mrs White's questions and do not have to cover all areas in the time allocated.

FURTHER INFORMATION

Mrs White is married and this is her third child. Her husband works away from home a lot of the time. There is no family history of CF.

This station assesses your ability to communicate appropriate, factually correct information in an effective way within the emotional context of the clinical setting:

- **Communication Two**

This is a 9-minute station consisting of spoken interaction. You will have up to 2 minutes before the start of the station to read this sheet and prepare yourself. You may make notes on the paper provided.

When the bell sounds you will be invited into the examination room. Please take this instruction sheet with you. The examiner will not ask questions during the 9 minutes but will warn you when you have approximately 2 minutes left.

You are not required to examine a patient.

The encounter should be focused on the task; you will be penalised for asking irrelevant questions or providing superfluous information. You will be marked on your ability to communicate, not the speed with which you convey information. You may not have time to complete the communication.

SETTING

You are a paediatric SpR working on the neonatal unit.

SCENARIO

The nurses have asked you to talk to the mother of James about discharge arrangements. He is due to go home tomorrow but you are expecting the delivery of premature triplets today and his space on the unit is needed.

BACKGROUND

James was born at 25 weeks' gestation. He is now 39 weeks' corrected gestation. He was ventilated for 2 weeks and required CPAP for a further month. He was out of oxygen by 34 weeks' corrected gestation. He had a right-sided IVH. He had a PDA, which was successfully closed with indomethacin. He was investigated for sepsis on two occasions. James required NG feeds for a prolonged period but has now successfully established breast feeds and is gaining weight.

He is the only child of his parents. His father works away from home a lot.

STATION 9

This station assesses your ability to take a focused history and explain to the parent your diagnosis or differential management plan:

- History-taking and Management planning

This is a 22-minute station of spoken interaction. You will have up to 4 minutes beforehand to prepare yourself. The scenario is below. Be aware that you should focus on the task given. You will be penalised for asking irrelevant questions or providing superfluous information. When the bell sounds you will be invited into the examination room. You will have 13 minutes with the patient (with a warning when you have 4 minutes left). You will then have a short period to reflect on the case while the patient leaves the room. You will then have 9 minutes with the examiner.

INFORMATION

You are the specialist registrar working in a district general hospital. You receive the following letter from a GP and are seeing the family in an outpatient clinic:

Dear Doctor

Re: Sumira Mussuamba DOB 9/12/1996

Sumira is an 8-year-old asylum seeker from Somalia who has been in the UK for 8 months with her mother and siblings. Sumira's father died during the conflict in Somalia.

I think Sumira had febrile convulsions as an infant and there is a family history of febrile convulsions.

Since moving to the UK Sumira has begun to have convulsions. They begin on the left side and become generalised. She is unresponsive and her eyes roll. She has been to A&E on one occasion but did not stay overnight.

Please could you see this child, who has recently joined my practice, for further management of her fits? I have commenced sodium valproate 400 mg bd.

Many thanks,
Dr Smith

How do you approach the history in this case?

DIAGNOSIS: DOWN'S SYNDROME WITH AVSD

Children with Down's syndrome are commonly utilised in exams as they may have multiple pathologies but are gifted with an extremely pleasant temperament. It is a syndrome you should know inside out and back to front.

This station is testing your ability to combine clinical findings from a variety of sources. You must be able to utilise your clinical skills to detect a murmur and provide the differentials: ventriculoseptal defect (VSD) or atrioventricular septal defect (AVSD). As the murmur is at the lower left sternal edge it is unlikely to be PS or AS. Realising this child has Down's syndrome then makes AVSD the most likely diagnosis because it is the most common cardiac defect in Down's syndrome.

You should have noted:

The apex was near the mid-axillary line and therefore this child has cardiomegaly.
The second heart sound is louder, indicating a degree of pulmonary hypertension.
The absence of a thrill makes an AVSD more likely (although if the VSD is severe the thrill may be absent and an AVSD may have a thrill).
No mention of a diastolic murmur but a diastolic flow murmur may well be present at the apex of lower left sternal edge.

The examiner will then further expect you to realise that not only must this lesion be repaired but also that Down's children have an increased risk of pulmonary hypertension so will have an earlier surgical intervention. You may pass this station for a correct description of the presenting feature but what will gain you the vital clear pass marks is the ability to apply your findings to this particular clinical scenario.

Immediate investigations are an ECG (biventricular hypertrophy) and CXR to assess the degree of cardiomegaly with an ECHO to define the extent of the anatomical defect. An ECHO can also estimate the pressure in the right ventricle (by calculating the Doppler measure pressure difference between the right and left ventricle and knowing the systemic pressure). However, evidence of severe pulmonary hypertension will require cardiac catheterisation to quantify the degree of pulmonary vascular resistance.

Treatment will involve diuretics but only surgery will be curative.
The following list should be well known to you.

CLASSIC FEATURES IN DOWN'S SYNDROME

Newborn

Frequent:

- Hypotonia
- Excess skin on nape of neck

- Slanted palpebral fissures
- Poor Moro reflex.

Common:

- Single palmar crease
- Accessory auricles
- Fifth finger clinodactyly
- Sandal gap of toes.

Head	Hands	Heart
Flat occiput	Fifth finger	AVSD
Epicanthic folds	Absence of middle phalanx	VSD
Brushfield's spots in iris	Single crease	PDA
Protruding tongue	Distal axial triradius	Tetralogy of Fallot
Small ears	Broad appearance	Increased risk of
	Hyperextensible	pulmonary vascular
		disease

COMMON ASSOCIATIONS OF DOWN'S SYNDROME

A Alzheimer's

T Thyroid problems (hypothyroid)
R Respiratory infections
I Instable atlanto-axial joint
S Small bowel atresia
O Otitis media
M Mental retardation
Y Y chromosome (males) – infertile

C Cataracts
H Hirschsprung's
I Eye problems (squint and cataract)
L Leukaemia
D Duodenal atresia

REMINDER

There does seem to be a degree of discrepancy in the definition of atrial septal defects (ASDs), ostium primum or secundum defects and atrioventricular defects in different textbooks.

A quick review of the anatomy may be helpful (see Fig. 1).

An ASD, a hole between the atria as most medical students learn it, can be referred to as an ostium secundum defect and occur at the site of the fossa ovalis.

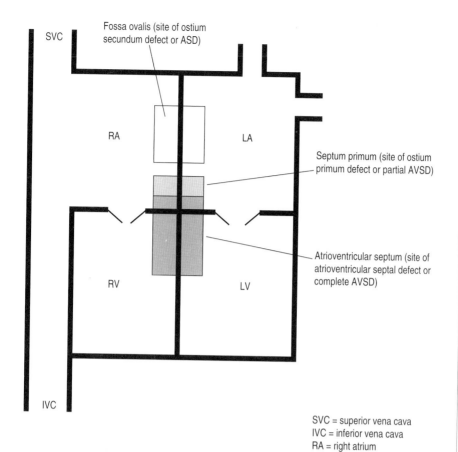

Figure 1 Diagram of the heart showing the sites of ASD, partial AVSD and complete AVSD

SVC = superior vena cava
IVC = inferior vena cava
RA = right atrium
RV = right ventricle
LA = left atrium

Lesions can also be inferior to the site of the ostium secundum and just touch the upper part of the ventricular septum. This is called an ostium primum ASD or may be referred to as an incomplete AVSD. Although the ventricular septum is intact, there are invariably abnormalities of the atrioventricular valves (often a mitral valve cleft).

A complete VSD involves the ventricular septum and allows communication of all four chambers of the heart. This is the commonest lesion in children with Down's syndrome.

CAN YOU …

List the common presenting features of Down's syndrome?

Ostium primum partial (AVSD)	Ostium secundum (ASD)
Soft ejection systolic murmur at left second intercostal area	Soft ejection systolic murmur at left second intercostal area
May have murmur at apex secondary to mitral regurgitation	
Left axis deviation	Right axis deviation
Partial right bundle branch block	Partial right bundle branch block

COMMENTS ON STATION 2

DIAGNOSIS: GLYCOGEN STORAGE DISORDER

This child has a glycogen storage disorder (GSD) which, if your revision is going very well, you will know is most likely to be von Gierke's disease (GSD type 1). If you are lucky enough to have seen a child with this condition and are able to recognise 'doll's face facies' then in the real exam this station may be much easier. Many classic facial appearances, the prominent forehead of Alagille's syndrome, the saddle-shaped nose of fetal alcohol syndrome and the triangular appearance of Russell–Silver syndrome will not be readily apparent to you in the exam. The examiner is not going to fail you for missing these features (although it would be difficult to justify missing a Down's syndrome unless the appearance was very subtle). It is much more important to pick up the hard clinical signs and put them in their correct context rather than be a good syndrome spotter. This child has impressive hepatomegaly without the presence of splenomegaly. The only evidence of chronic liver disease is the bruising, but overt liver failure seems unlikely given the absence of jaundice (and the child's presence in the exam!). If you had not thought of storage diseases an appropriate response would be:

> 'This child shows evidence of poor growth, a tendency to bruise either by platelet or clotting factor deficiency and/or dysfunction and gross hepatomegaly. The absence of splenomegaly reduces the likelihood of a myeloproliferative disorder or red blood cell defect. I need to confirm this is not right heart failure but I see no overt evidence of cardiorespiratory distress. My primary investigations would be based on looking for problems with liver metabolism, function or structure.'

Once you are focused on the liver, hopefully your list of causes of hepatomegaly will jump out at you!

Some key features of the glycogen storage disorders are worth knowing as they are stable patients with good signs, making them popular exam patients. It is worth looking at the size of the patient's tongue as macroglossia is associated with Pompe's disease (GSD type 2). Asking the

Hepatomegaly alone	Splenomegaly alone	Hepatosplenomegaly
Glycogen storage disorders Heart failure Galactosaemia Wilson's disease	Portal hypertension Red blood cell defect (hereditary spherocytosis, sickle cell anaemia) Chronic ITP	Myeloproliferative disorder Mucopolysaccharidoses α_1-Antitrypsin deficiency

mother if Sarah has a problem with her sugar levels should clinch the diagnosis of GSD.

The underlying problem for glycogen storage disorders is the inability to break down glycogen into a useful substrate for energy. Although there are over 10 known types it is more useful to divide them into those which affect muscle or those affecting the liver or those affecting both.

Type	Name	Organ affected	Special features
1	Von Gierke's	Liver	Most common May present as asymptomatic hepatomegaly Short individuals May have large kidneys Overnight feeds Corn starch used in older children Increased risk of hepatoma
2	Pompe's	Muscle	Three types (infantile form most common) Infant form results in heart failure before 12 months of age Gross weakness and floppiness without muscle wasting Macroglossia
3	Cori's	Muscle/liver	Massive hepatomegaly Muscle weakness common Frequent feedings and high protein diet
4	Anderson's	Liver/muscle	Progressive cirrhosis Presents as failure to thrive
5	McArdle's	Muscle	Muscle cramps post-exercise Risk of myoglobinuria and renal failure post-heavy exercise

CAN YOU …

Name the common causes of macroglossia?

- Congenital hypothyroidism
- Beckwith–Wiedemann syndrome
- Pompe's GSD
- Mucopolysaccharidoses

Down's syndrome is not true macroglossia – the tongue protrudes forward in a relatively small mouth

COMMENTS ON STATION 3

DIAGNOSIS: SPINA BIFIDA

This child has spina bifida and must have a lesion below L2 and possibly commencing as low down as L5. This is a difficult case because it requires you to examine and think at the same time. Candidates come unstuck in neurological cases because they are so concerned about getting the examination correct they completely ignore the findings they have obtained. You must be able to perform a neurological exam without having to worry about what to do next. It must just come naturally. In the stress of the exam you will forget to do something or realise you have no idea which muscle was weak. You should not be examined by a paediatric neurologist, although you should make sure you are taught by one.

> 'This child has had a surgical repair of a lumbosacral lesion, presumably a meningocele or meningomyelocele. In light of this finding I elected to examine the lower limbs to define the level of the lesion. I will also need to examine the head, looking in particular for any evidence of hydrocephalus, as up to 90% of children with spina bifida may have an Arnold–Chiari malformation. On examination the child was not particularly wasted and the most obvious defect was the absence of hip extension, plantar flexion and ankle reflex. As I noted some spontaneous knee extension the lesion is likely to spare L3 and perhaps L4. I need to examine the anus to complete my lower limb examination.'

There is a degree of difference in textbooks about specific myotomes and reflex roots which can make revision difficult. The suggested levels worked for the author but may differ slightly from other books. The important thing is not to be too precise about the level but be very consistent with your observations and findings.

There are many peripheral issues in spina bifida which must be addressed, and may be part of a communication or history-taking station.

Medical	Functional	Social
Hydrocephalus (presence of shunt, CSF infection)	Mobility (need for wheelchair or callipers)	Education (need for special class or school if intellectual impairment)
Orthopaedics (callipers, contracture release)	Incontinence (use of anticholinergics)	Development
Ulcers (pressure sores)	MDT involvement (Physio/OT)	Adolescent issues
UTIs (increased risk of reflux)		
Scoliosis/kyphosis		
Eyes (ambylopia secondary to squint)		

REFLEXES

Triceps: C7,8
Biceps: C5,6
Knee: L3,4
Ankle: S1,2

Remember Jendrassik's manoeuvre. Just before the reflex is elicited the child should be asked to perform an action to produce muscle tension: 'Screw up your face', 'Pull your locked hands away from each other', 'Squeeze your fists', etc. (see Fig. 2).

Dermatome: upper		Dermatome: lower	
Lateral surface upper arm	C5	Inguinal region	L1
Tip of thumb	C6	Medial surface upper thigh	L2
Web between fingers	C7	Medial surface lower thigh	L3
Tip of little finger	C8	Medial surface lower leg	L4
Medial surface lower arm	T1	Lateral surface lower leg	L5
Medial surface upper arm	T2	Lateral surface of foot	S1
		Medial surface upper calf	S2
		Medial surface inner thigh	S3
		Perianal	S4

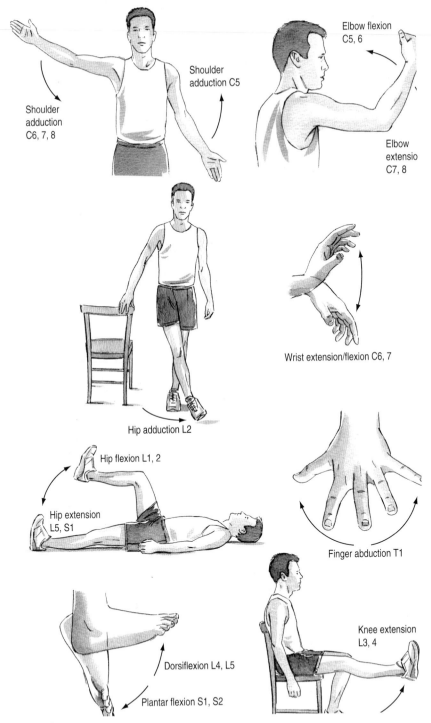

Figure 2

DIAGNOSIS: MARFAN'S SYNDROME

A station with the potential for so many positive clinical findings is an ideal examination case but the candidate must be careful to remember them all when presenting in the heat of the moment. The findings of arachnodactyly, tall height and scoliosis should make you consider whether she has Marfan's syndrome. Had you examined her oropharynx you would have noted a high-arched palate. The degree of kyphoscoliosis or chest wall deformity may produce problems in respiratory function resulting in a picture of restrictive lung disease.

Marfan's syndrome should be easily recognisable and could appear in the cardiac, respiratory or 'other' stations. We would expect that the child would usually be a teenager.

	Tips
Genetics	Autosomal dominant with variable expression, chromosome 15
Features	Skeletal: arachnodactyly Tall stature Lower segment > upper segment Arm span > height Scoliosis High-arched palate Joint hypermobility Sternberg's sign (can adduct thumb across palm) CVS: aortic dissection Mitral valve prolapse RS: pneumothorax Eyes: lens dislocation
Management	Regular ECHO and BP measurement. Ocular examination Prognosis affected by cardiac lesion
Differential	Homocysteinuria: thrombosis, learning difficulties, osteoporosis and homocysteine in urine Klinefelter's syndrome Acromegaly (rare) In the following conditions the final adult height is usually normal despite a greater rate of growth as a child: Soto's syndrome Beckwith–Wiedemann syndrome Hyperthyroidism Precocious puberty Familial tall stature is the commonest cause of tall stature, although the examiners much prefer showing children with signs!

CAN YOU …

Describe the differences between Marfan's syndrome and homocystinuria?

Although phenotypically similar, the most notable differences are the presence of homocystine in the urine and the absence of intellectual difficulty in homocystinuria. Most candidates only remember that there are differences in the direction of lens subluxation. It may be that you are confident in remembering the difference, but some authorities are not convinced about this method of differentiating the conditions. The dislocation would also have to be quite marked in order to correctly document the direction.

- *Marfan's*: up and out
- *Homocystinuria*: down and cyst**IN**uria

COMMENTS ON STATION 5

DIAGNOSIS: THYROID SWELLING

There is a classic medical school urban myth where a student in his final-year exam becomes very flustered when asked to examine the thyroid gland of a young child. Having sweated, pontificated and prodded hopelessly at the front of the child's neck the examiner comments that there is a glass of water on the side table if that would be helpful. The student, grateful for the examiner's intervention, drinks the glass of water himself.

Have you examined a thyroid gland or assessed thyroid status as part of your revision? It is very easily overlooked as thyroid presentations are uncommon on acute takes, generally being managed in outpatient clinics. However, patients are easily available, generally well and have hard clinical signs.

Thyroid stations involve examination of the gland itself and assessment of the thyroid status. There are then a number of 'classic' questions which you will be expected to ask the parents and/or child.

THYROID EYE DISEASE

Although not universally present, there are simple techniques to look for the classic features of hyperthyroid eye disease:

- *Exophthalmos*: An abnormal protrusion of the eyeball. Some texts interchange the term for proptosis, others preferring to use exophthalmos for an endocrinologically caused protrusion. Looking from above the child's head for a forward eye bulge is not a terribly objective exam but it is obvious to the examiner what you are trying to do.
- *Lid retraction*: The sclera above the iris is visible at rest. If not present, test for lid lag.
- *Lid lag*: Ask the child to follow a horizontally placed finger up and down. If you are able to see the sclera above the iris on downward gaze this sign is positive.
- *External ophthalmoplegia*: Uncommonly the lateral or superior rectus muscles may be affected.

Examination

General appearance	Must ask for weight and height Asking for height velocity shows insight into condition Pendred's syndrome is a goitre (not necessarily hypothyroidism) and hearing loss. Look for hearing aid A horizontal necklace scar indicates a thyroidectomy (so check voice for hoarseness) Ask about pubertal staging
Inspection	Ask the child to take a drink – the gland should rise on swallowing Ask the child to stick his/her tongue out – a thyroglossal cyst will rise with this procedure
Palpation	Palpate from behind the child (and again while they drink) As with all lumps: • Shape • Size • Softness • Surface (one or multiple lumps)
Other gland examination	Local lymphadenopathy Percuss sternum and palpate suprasternal notch for retrosternal extension Auscultate the murmur for a bruit
Thyroid status (head to toe)	**Hypothyroid** Swollen eyes with eyebrow loss Thin, dry hair and skin Bradycardic Cool peripheries Hyporeflexic	**Hyperthyroid** Classic eye signs May have goitre bruit Tachycardic Warm, sweaty hands Proximal muscle weakness Wide pulse pressure

History

Hypothyroid	Hyperthyroid
Do teachers describe your child as an attentive pupil? Has school performance deteriorated after treatment? Has you child had any problems with constipation? Does your child feel the cold more than their siblings? Has you child started to gain weight recently? Has your child had any difficulty walking? (slipped upper femoral epiphysis)	Does you child have problems sleeping? Has you child ever complained of palpitations? Has your child become emotionally labile? How is your child performing at school?

Hypothyroid child

- Autoimmune (increased incidence in girls)
- Family history may be present
- Associated with diabetes mellitus
- T4 low and TSH high at diagnosis
- Treat with T4
- Must monitor levels of T4 and TSH

Hyperthyroid child:

- Graves' disease (productions of antithyroid antibodies)
- Adolescent girls
- HLA DR3/B8
- TSH low and T4 high at diagnosis
- TSH receptor-stimulating antibodies can be shown to regress on remission
- Treat with carbimazole over 2-year period, although relapse rate is high
- Propranolol can be used for acute symptoms
- Steroid for eye disease
- May need (sub)total thyroidectomy
- May become subsequently hypothyroid

REMINDER

Other anterior neck swellings

Midline	Lateral
Thyroglossal cyst	Lymphadenopathy (primary or secondary)
Epidermoid cyst	Cystic hygroma
	Branchial cyst
	Sternomastoid 'tumour' (neonatal)

COMMENTS ON STATION 6

DIAGNOSIS: EX 27-WEEK NEONATAL GRADUATE

By the time you have introduced yourself to the examiner, said hello to mum and overcome the nausea you may be feeling, a good minute will have passed. The examiner is certainly going to want to ask you questions, especially if things are going badly, so you may only have 5 minutes to actually examine the patient. Unless you are very lucky your developmental examination is unlikely to be systematic and you can certainly not predict how long it will take you to examine each of the different categories. You must therefore accept that by the time you come to present your findings to the examiner you may not have all the information you would wish.

It has been emphasised that knowledge of your milestones is paramount and your recall must be a reflex. You must see each particular movement, noise or skill a child makes as an age. This is very easy to practise. Walk around any supermarket on a weekend afternoon and guess the ages of children. I do not recommend asking the parents how old their child actually is as someone might call the police! You will quickly realise what knowledge you have to hand and what you can't remember.

This child has a developmental age of at least 6 months:

Sits without support
Rolls front to back
Palmar grasp
Responds to sounds
No stranger anxiety

and shows some features of a 9-month-old:

Looks for fallen object
Rolls back to front

but not others:

Pulls to stand
Developing pincer grip

and is obviously not the developmental equivalent of a 1-year-old child. There are many potential reasons for this but note the delay is spread across all four developmental fields. Realising that the child is small, plagiocephalic and has neonatal scars makes prematurity the most likely cause.

The causes of developmental delay are numerous but can be categorised in order to provide a framework for an answer:

Cause of developmental delay	Examples
Congenital/syndromic	Down's syndrome
Central neurological	Isolated motor delays (e.g. the bottom shuffler)
Idiopathic mental retardation	
Peripheral neurological	Muscular dystrophy, spinal muscular atrophy
Familial	
Environmental/social	Parental neglect Malnourished

The approach to the assessment of developmentally delayed children is a lengthy process (much like failure to thrive) and again requires a similar framework. It is important to try not to learn a list of investigations but realise there are different areas which may be assessed. Yes, it may be worth looking for azurophilic dispersed hypergranulation of polymorphonuclear cells (neuronal ceroid lipofuscinosis) but not if you haven't taken a pregnancy history first.

It is vital in the history to have a good documentation of the timeline of growth and development. A good history that skills have been lost raises the possibility that the child has a neurodegenerative or metabolic condition, whereas the failure to obtain skills may represent a primary neurological condition.

ASSESSMENT OF DEVELOPMENTAL DELAY

History
Pregnancy:

- Complications
- Fetal growth
- Gestational age at birth
- Perinatal complications

Neonatal:

- Early growth
- Feeding history

Infancy:

- Developmental milestones
- Specific abnormalities:
  - Failure to thrive
  - Seizures
  - Loss of skills

Family:

- Previously affected children
- Medical/psychiatric history of parents
- Consanguinity

Social:

- Education (of parents and child)
- Who lives at home?
- Social service involvement
- Who is the main carer?

Medical:

- Is a paediatrician involved?
- Is a health visitor involved?
- Any known medical problems?

The above digresses from the clinical remit of the developmental station but you may well be asked how you would investigate developmental delay. Your assessment should be concluded by a thorough physical exam (including evidence of dysmorphology) – and remember to measure growth parameters!

Investigations should be tailored to the history and not a blind repetition of all the blood tests you know.

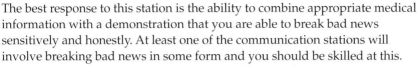
The best response to this station is the ability to combine appropriate medical information with a demonstration that you are able to break bad news sensitively and honestly. At least one of the communication stations will involve breaking bad news in some form and you should be skilled at this.

These tips for 'breaking bad news' should be very familiar to you:

Setting

- Set aside time
- Quiet setting
  - Side room; hand bleep over to a colleague to avoid disturbance
- Have an accompanying nurse and relative present
  - If not, offer to meet them at a later stage
- Introduce yourself fully.

Communication

- Establish what the patient knows
- Give information clearly and simply
- Use active listening – pauses, 'Umm', 'yes', etc.
- Invite and answer questions
- Review family's support network
- Give appropriate hope.

Conclusion

- Summarise
- Arrange further meeting
- Offer to meet family members.

You can show the examiner that you know how to set the scene for such an interview by using stock sentences such as:

'I have given my bleep to my colleague so that we will not be disturbed.'

'If your husband would like to talk to me about this, I will be happy to meet with him to explain.'

When thinking about how you will discuss a diagnosis such as cystic fibrosis with a family in the exam, it is recommended to read information leaflets from associated organisations – they are excellent for tips on how to describe illness in 'layman's' terms and for answering common questions.

Before you enter the consultation, consider which aspects of the disease you wish to cover. Keep things relatively simple and remember that the parents will only retain small amounts of the information given. They will also have prepared questions to ask in the exam!

For this consultation we would include:

- Result of Guthrie
- Description of CF

- Further investigations needed to make diagnosis
- Initial management if confirmed to have CF.

A possible consultation may go in the following way:

'We have received the results of Hayley's Guthrie heel-prick test. This test screens babies for a variety of illnesses that we can identify early on so that we can begin treatment. The test suggests that Hayley may have cystic fibrosis. [Pause] Do you know anything about CF? …

'CF is an inherited disease which mainly affects the lungs and digestive system. There is a fault in mucus production and the mucus in CF patients is thick and prone to infection. Not all children are affected to the same extent.

'We need to do some further tests to confirm whether Hayley has CF. We would like to take some blood for genetic testing and a "sweat test" to see how salty Hayley's sweat is.

'If these tests confirm that Hayley has CF she will need to be referred to the nearest hospital which manages CF. We will be able to monitor her growth and to try and prevent infections with antibiotics and physiotherapy.'

This is a huge diagnosis to give and you potentially may spend more time answering questions than covering all the above points. The above answer doesn't even touch on potential parental concerns of genetics and the 'it's all my fault' response.

TESTS ON GUTHRIE CARD (POTENTIALLY – NOT ALL CENTRES OFFER ALL TESTS)

- Hypothyroidism
- PKU
- Cystic fibrosis
- Sickle cell disease/thalassaemia
- Very-long-chain fatty acid (VLCFA) and medium-chain fatty acid (MCFA) defects

SWEAT TESTS

CF causes elevated Na and Cl in sweat. A level of Na and CL $> 60\,\text{mEq/L}$ is abnormal and $40\text{–}60\,\text{mEq/L}$ is borderline.

Indications

- Abnormal neonatal screening (should not be performed at <1 week of age)
- Meconium ileus
- Suggestive symptoms, e.g. FTT, repeated chest infections, prolonged diarrhoea

Techniques

Technique involves quantitative pilocarpine iontophoresis. Two discs are placed on to cleaned skin a few inches apart and an electric current is passed between them. The sweat produced is collected on a paper disc or a macro-duct. It takes up to 30 minutes to collect enough sweat (100 mg of sweat is needed). The sodium and chloride are measured in the lab.

COMMENTS ON STATION 8

The best scenario you can hope for will be about a topic that you encounter in everyday practice and feel confident discussing. The above situation may have occurred in your unit (although in real practice this child would be more effectively managed in transitional care). The examiners are looking for your ability to communicate effectively, empathically and to listen constructively regardless of the situation you are placed in. Perhaps, in this situation, you may get more time in the exam to prepare yourself than you would do in your place of work! The minutes before you go into the room are therefore vital in outlining the structure of the conversation in your head.

When a candidate read this type of question in the exam, they thought the mother had been informed about the bed shortage and need for discharge on that day and had planned a conversation about feeding, family care follow-up, immunisations, etc. It quickly became clear that the news needed breaking first – and a quick recovery was needed!

Here is a possible outline for this conversation:

- Introduce yourself and confirm the name of parent.
- Ask if they wish to have a friend/relative present.
- Try to make the suggestion that you have a nurse with you in the room (they will be imaginary).
- Say that you will not be interrupted during the consultation.
- Offer the opportunity for them to ask questions at any time.
- Recap briefly on James's progress to date on the unit and reiterate how well he is now doing with feeding and growing.
- Ask what his mother understands about the discharge arrangements.
- Introduce the idea of discharge a day early and why this has become necessary.
- Review the mother's concerns around discharge and home support network.
- Decide whether discharge that day is possible.
- Review general follow-up, immunisations and sources of help.
- Agree a plan.
- Summarise.
- Give opportunity for questions.

In the role-player's information, the mother was not prepared for discharge that day as her husband was away on business. It may therefore be decided that she would room-in that night on the unit and be discharged the following day. She will have had many questions about follow-up and James's future health.

COMMENTS ON STATION 9

This station re-emphasises the importance of seeing new referrals in general paediatric outpatient clinics. You must have a scheme for taking a thorough history without missing important points specific to seizures.

When taking a history of a first fit you must include:

- Birth history (any neonatal fits)
- Development (especially delay in first 2 years of life)
- Did the child have febrile convulsions?
- Any current medical therapy?
- Any history suggestive of a cardiac cause?
- Description of convulsion, ideally from an eye-witness account:
  - Time of day
  - Preceding events
  - Any aura (if old enough to describe)
  - Length of convulsion
  - Type of convulsion
  - Responsiveness during convulsion
  - Length of post-ictal period
- Management of fits (what do parents do?)
- Frequency
- Family history
- Patient and child understanding and concerns.

The scenario from the letter is very open-ended: a number of different types of fit are possible (see table).

The history will be more important than the diagnosis. The examiner will be looking for you to have asked all the appropriate questions without being sidetracked by the response of the child or parent. In particular, you should not put words into the patient's mouth or assume a family's understanding of the meaning of medical terminology. For example:

'So the twitching movement started in your child's face and then spread to their arms and legs?' is obviously suggestive compared to *'What happened after the facial twitching?'*

'Was your child incontinent?', 'Was your child cyanotic?', '... and your child was unconscious?' assumes a good command of English (note the background of the patients in the scenario). I have seen doctors ask about 'cyanosis' when questioning parents. It is not intentional but very easy to do when under pressure. If the answers are simply nodded replies then you may find yourself assuming things that never happened.

When questioned about her management of her daughter's seizure it becomes apparent that cold water is splashed on her until she stops. Because the seizures always stop her mother has assumed that this is the correct treatment!

Seizure	Features
Simple partial	Any part of body May spread to become generalised Often secondary to structural defect Focal spikes or slow wave in affected area
Benign partial (Rolandic) EEG: centrotemporal spikes	Partial, which may progress to generalised Often commences in face and tongue (parents hear gargling noise from bedroom) Often nocturnal or early morning Remits in adolescence
Myoclonic – akinetic	Violent contractions of muscle groups. May throw patients to the side Minimal or no loss of consciousness Usually evidence/history of brain neurone damage Lennox–Gastaut if associated with mental retardation
Juvenile myoclonic EEG: 4–7 Hz spike wave activity	Early-morning myoclonic jerks (typically of head and neck) Associated with generalised tonic–clonic seizures
Absence EEG: three-per-second spike wave activity	Vacant episodes up to 10 seconds 'Automatisms' of face No aura or post-ictal confusion
Generalised tonic–clonic EEG: bilaterally synchronous multiple high-voltage spikes	Loss of consciousness Often preceded by aura or cry May have bladder incontinence or tongue biting
Temporal lobe	Clinical features similar to absence seizures (staring, odd facial expressions and fidgeting hand movements) However, may have aura, last longer (30–60 seconds) and autonomic disturbance

Management may include medical treatment but more importantly a thorough explanation of acute management of the seizure (if only to place the child in the recovery position).

The investigation of convulsions depends on the history and frequency of fits. Often a single tonic–clonic convulsion is not investigated (5% of children will have a fit at some point in their lives). A third of children with a single afebrile convulsion will not have a further episode.

All children must have:

- A thorough neurological examination including fundoscopy
- Blood glucose with every prolonged fit which presents to hospital
- Head circumference measurement
- Blood pressure measurement.

Units differ on the initial blood tests and investigations required but after two or more afebrile convulsions consider:

- Full blood count, urea and electrolytes, calcium, magnesium
- EEG
- ECG and CXR if evidence of cardiac cause
- Explanation of fits and emergency first aid treatment (if not offered at initial presentation)
- UV (Wood's) light to look for ash leaf depigmentation (tuberous sclerois).

For seizures of a typical nature brain imaging is not required; however, bear in mind that cranial ultrasound may be used in those whose fontanelle has not closed. Children with focal seizures, abnormal neurology and developmental delay will need consideration of a CT or MRI.

Generally sodium valproate is used to treat generalised convulsions and carbamazepine to treat simple or complex partial seizures. It would be unusual for a first-year registrar to commence anti-epileptic medication for a newly diagnosed epileptic without the supervision of a consultant. Therefore, it is more important to know common features of anti-epileptic medications rather than the latest research on their efficacy.

Side effects of most anti-epileptic medication:

- Weight gain (this seems to be of most importance to teenage girls)
- Nausea and vomiting
- Drowsiness.

Toxic effects include ataxia, confusion, dysarthria and nystagmus.

An unexplained rash should prompt medical review and cessation of medication.

Lastly it is easy to forget some of the social effects epilepsy may have. Children should not cycle in busy traffic or swim unsupervised. For the young adult, they should be aware they must be seizure free for a year in order to be able to drive.

Circuit C

STATION 1

This station assesses your ability to elicit clinical signs:

- **CVS**

This is a 9-minute station of clinical interaction. You will have up to 4 minutes beforehand to prepare yourself. No additional information will be given or is necessary before commencing the station. When the bell sounds you will be invited into the examination room.

INTRODUCTION

On entering the station you are presented with a girl approximately 9 years old. You are told, 'A GP has referred this child because he thinks she has a heart murmur. What do you think?'.

CLINICAL SCENARIO

The girl is comfortable at rest. You commence your routine cardiovascular examination. There are no abnormalities until you commence auscultation of the precordium. You hear a systolic murmur at the lower left sternal edge but also, and if not louder, in the aortic and pulmonary areas. You are uncertain as to whether this is an ejection systolic or pansystolic murmur. You feel a thrill in the suprasternal notch. You find no evidence of heart failure and can find no scars.

Where must you examine in order to clinch your diagnosis?

If this is positive what else will you look at?

Which syndromes are linked to this cardiac abnormality?

This station assesses your ability to elicit clinical signs:
- **Abdo/Other**

INTRODUCTION

On entering the station you are given the instruction, 'Please examine this 16-year-old boy's abdominal system, paying close attention to his nutritional status. Why do you think he has a scar?'.

CLINICAL SCENARIO

The boy looks smaller than you would expect for his age and has a gaunt appearance. Peripheral examination potentially shows some wasting of the hands, his conjunctivae are pale but his mouth is free from ulcers. You note that his muscle bulk looks reduced and offer to test this. There is a large laparotomy scar across his stomach but apart from some mild tenderness in the left iliac fossa abdominal examination is unremarkable.

How do you test his muscle bulk?

What else will you ask for and examine?

How do you present this patient?

STATION 3

This station assesses your ability to elicit clinical signs:
- **Neurological**

This is a 9-minute station of clinical interaction. You will have up to 4 minutes beforehand to prepare yourself. No additional information will be given or is necessary before commencing the station. When the bell sounds you will be invited into the examination room.

INTRODUCTION

On entering the station you are presented with an African girl approximately 10 years old with an obvious movement disorder. You are asked to comment on her appearance and the abnormal movements.

CLINICAL SCENARIO

The child appears agitated and has persistent jerking movements of her arms. They move in an uncoordinated fashion, obviously to the girl's distress. She is unable to keep her hands held together. Occasionally she demonstrates some facial grimacing.

How will you approach your examination?

What important differentials should you be aware of?

You are told she was a normal child 3 months ago and there is no family history of metabolic or neurological disorder. What investigations would you consider?

STATION 4

This station assesses your ability to elicit clinical signs:
- **Respiratory/Other**

This is a 9-minute station of clinical interaction. You will have up to 4 minutes beforehand to prepare yourself. No additional information will be given or is necessary before commencing the station. When the bell sounds you will be invited into the examination room.

INTRODUCTION

On entering the room you are presented with a child approximately 5 years old. You are asked to examine his respiratory system to discover why he is coughing so much.

CLINICAL SCENARIO

The child is sitting on his mother's knee. You ask to move him to the examining couch but his mother is uncertain as to whether he will cooperate. You explain that you would like at least to try. As soon as he is lifted towards the bed he starts crying. You quickly ask the mother to sit him on her lap and explain to the examiner that it may be easier to examine the child while he is settled.

On inspection he has a respiratory rate of 35 but no obvious recession. He has no scars, does not look cyanosed or anaemic but does cough during the examination. At one point he produces some mucky sputum.

While sitting on his mother's lap he lets you examine him. His chest is not overtly hyperexpanded and there is good air entry, apart from the right base which has reduced air entry with multiple crackles and creps. The percussion note at this point is equivocal. The left side of his chest sounds clear.

Of interest, he has a cannula in his left hand. There is no oxygen in the room.

What else do you need to know to make your diagnosis?

STATION 5

This station assesses your ability to elicit clinical signs:
- **Other**

This is a 9-minute station of clinical interaction. You will have up to 4 minutes beforehand to prepare yourself. No additional information will be given or is necessary before commencing the station. When the bell sounds you will be invited into the examination room.

INTRODUCTION

On entering the room you are presented with a child approximately 2 years old. You are asked to comment on any striking features and discuss how this might relate to the child's anaemia.

CLINICAL SCENARIO

On general inspection the child is pale and looks small for his age. He is playing with a toy in his mother's arms and you notice an abnormality to his right hand. On closer inspection he appears to have two thumbs but both are hypoplastic. The more proximal lacks a distal phalangeal segment and the distal is attached by only a small piece of skin (see Fig. 3).

What more do you want to examine in his upper limbs?

After presenting your findings, which other parts of the body will you examine?

Just before presenting your overall findings you notice some café-au-lait spots on the child's chest. What could the diagnosis be?

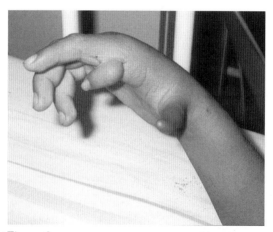

Figure 3

This station assesses your ability to assess specifically requested areas in a child with a developmental problem:

- Development

This is a 9-minute station of clinical interaction. You will have up to 4 minutes beforehand to prepare yourself. No additional information will be given or is necessary before commencing the station. When the bell sounds you will be invited into the examination room.

INTRODUCTION

You are informed that you are to assess this child's speech and language.

CLINICAL SCENARIO

A child about 5 years old is playing with a ball in the centre of the room. You notice immediately that he has hemifacial hypoplasia. His left eye, cheek and ear are deformed. His external auditory meatus is nearly entirely absent on the affected side, with his eye present but obstructed on the lateral aspect by overlying skin. His mandible is not well formed and causes his mouth to appear lopsided.

How do you assess his hearing?

Will the dysmorphism affect how you approach this case?

What can a 5-year-old child do?

STATION 7

This station assesses your ability to communicate appropriate, factually correct information in an effective way within the emotional context of the clinical setting:

- **Communication One**

This is a 9-minute station consisting of spoken interaction. You will have up to 2 minutes before the start of the station to read this sheet and prepare yourself. You may make notes on the paper provided.

When the bell sounds you will be invited into the examination room. Please take this instruction sheet with you. The examiner will not ask questions during the 9 minutes but will warn you when you have approximately 2 minutes left.

You are not required to examine a patient.

The encounter should be focused on the task; you will be penalised for asking irrelevant questions or providing superfluous information. You will be marked on your ability to communicate, not the speed with which you convey information. You may not have time to complete the communication.

SETTING

You are a specialist registrar working at a district general hospital which has a large number of medical students.

SCENARIO

It is the start of the new academic year and the next intake of paediatric medical students have just started their attachment. All the students are to undergo training in basic life support (airway, breathing and circulation) of an infant. You are to instruct Robert in how to manage a 2-year-old child who is not breathing and does not have a pulse. You may not complete the task in 9 minutes but you should teach in a systematic manner, ensuring Robert understands the tasks he must perform and that he performs them correctly. A mannequin with appropriate aids has been provided.

The scenario is that Robert finds this child in the hospital car park. He is not in danger and is able to send for help. He must provide basic life support until the paediatric crash team arrive.

This station assesses your ability to communicate appropriate, factually correct information in an effective way within the emotional context of the clinical setting:

- **Communication Two**

This is a 9-minute station consisting of spoken interaction. You will have up to 2 minutes before the start of the station to read this sheet and prepare yourself. You may make notes on the paper provided.

When the bell sounds you will be invited into the examination room. Please take this instruction sheet with you. The examiner will not ask questions during the 9 minutes but will warn you when you have approximately 2 minutes left.

You are not required to examine a patient.

The encounter should be focused on the task; you will be penalised for asking irrelevant questions or providing superfluous information. You will be marked on your ability to communicate, not the speed with which you convey information. You may not have time to complete the communication.

SETTING

You are a specialist registrar in a busy paediatric intensive care unit.

SCENARIO

Stephanie, a 5-year-old girl, was involved in a high-impact road traffic accident and has been on your unit for 8 days. She has suffered severe brain injury and is making no respiratory or neurological effort. A brain stem death test is to be performed by the consultant shortly after a long discussion with the parents. Stephanie's brother, Mark, who is 18, has been asking questions about the test and what it means. Her parents have asked for a doctor to speak to him as they feel too traumatised. The consultant asks you to speak to Mark.

BACKGROUND

Stephanie was a previously healthy girl who was hit by a car while crossing the road. Mark has only just arrived on the unit, having had to return from holiday. He is about to go to university to study law. He is unsure what brain stem death is and why the doctors can't leave her on the ventilator until her head is better and she wakes up. He is obviously extremely upset at not having been able to come home earlier.

Please sensitively discuss with Mark why you are performing a brain stem death test and what this might involve. You do not need to talk about Stephanie's management previously. The brain stem will show brain stem death. There will be no chance of recovery.

STATION 9

This station assesses your ability to take a focused history and explain to the parent your diagnosis or differential management plan:

- History-taking and Management planning

This is a 22-minute station of spoken interaction. You will have up to 4 minutes beforehand to prepare yourself. The scenario is below. Be aware that you should focus on the task given. You will be penalised for asking irrelevant questions or providing superfluous information. When the bell sounds you will be invited into the examination room. You will have 13 minutes with the patient (with a warning when you have 4 minutes left). You will then have a short period to reflect on the case while the patient leaves the room. You will then have 9 minutes with the examiner.

INFORMATION

You are a specialist registrar working in an outpatient clinic in a general district hospital. You receive the following letter from a GP:

Dear Doctor

Re: Steven 15 years

Thank you for seeing Steven, a type one diabetic who has been under my care for a number of years although I have only intermittently seen him since his last appointment at the diabetic clinic last year. Worryingly he was recently admitted in DKA with a poor record of his sugars in the preceding days. His mother has become concerned with his behaviour and is wondering whether his poor control recently is due to a change in his diabetes.

I would be very grateful for your help managing Steve's recent change in control.

BACKGROUND

Steven was diagnosed 6 years ago and has been on regular subcutaneous insulin since. His control has generally been very good and his last HbA1c measured at the diabetic review clinic last year was 6.5%.

Take a history from Steven and his mother and present your management plan to the examiner.

COMMENTS ON STATION 1

DIAGNOSIS: AORTIC STENOSIS

It would be nice if every child seen in the cardiovascular station has obvious signs and symptoms – but they don't. You may have a child with an unusual congenital heart defect whose abnormality is impossible to determine on clinical examination. So it is important to know what to rule out if your child has a murmur of indeterminate origin.

In this case you know the child has a systolic murmur without the presence of previous surgery or heart failure. What could this be?

- A ventricular septal defect which doesn't have a thrill
- Pulmonary stenosis
- Aortic stenosis
- Mitral regurgitation.

As the child is not cyanosed, and there are no scars, this child does not have an uncorrected cyanotic heart condition (tetralogy of Fallot, pulmonary atresia without a ventricular septal defect, etc.). Ventricular septal defect is a fair guess in a well child, although it is unusual to have a defect which isn't loudest at the lower left sternal edge. How do you rule out potentially more sinister defects? Pulmonary stenosis classically presents with an ejection systolic murmur maximal at the left sternal edge with an ejection click and split second heart sound. If all patients presented classically I think the exam would be a lot more fun! Fortunately aortic stenosis has a sign which cannot be present with other anomalies: a carotid thrill. The textbooks tell you a suprasternal thrill but pulmonary stenosis may also produce this. If a thrill is felt in the carotid region (and it is obvious, I promise!) then the murmur must be due to aortic stenosis. If you don't feel a thrill you are not much better off, as it could still be aortic stenosis, and all the other differentials! But it is an important negative.

If you ascertain the presence of a thrill then you should start feeling comfortable as there are a number of other features to start looking for, all relatively easy to learn.

Did you remember to ask the examiner to check peripheral pulses and perform a blood pressure?

REMINDERS

TURNER'S SYNDROME (full details can be found on p. 184)
45X (although mosaicism possible)
Proportional short stature
Cardiac disorders are the cause of increased mortality in this syndrome
Aortic coarctation most common cardiac defect
Dental malocclusion increased, so prophylaxis vital
Predisposition to keloid scar formation (child may have cardiac surgical scars)
Indication for using growth hormone (and consider using steroid to increase final height).

Aortic stenosis	Tips
Exam	Apex beat (do you always examine this?) may be displaced Suprasternal and carotid thrill Systolic murmur in aortic region and left sternal edge Have you felt for peripheral pulses? (Associated with coarctation) The slow rising pulse is a very difficult sign to elicit Have you listened to the back? (Not always helpful but there shouldn't be radiation, unlike in coarctation) A budding cardiology professor may pick up the diastolic murmur of aortic incompetence, which is more likely to occur post-surgery
Investigation	ECG normal in the well child but may show signs of left ventricular hypertrophy: • Tall R waves and inverted T waves in V5–V6 • CXR may show a prominent left ventricle • ECHO for diagnosis and management (assessing gradient)
Management	Generally a conservative approach with the guideline that a gradient of <60 mmHg across the valve requires no treatment. Surgical treatment is via balloon valvuloplasty and will have no obvious scar! Remember the murmur may remain post-surgery
Associated conditions	You should know and be able to quickly recite associations with: • Turner's syndrome • Williams' syndrome • Coarctation of the aorta

Oestrogen therapy to allow development of secondary sexual characteristics.

WILLIAMS' SYNDROME (also see p. 37)
Microdeletion chromosome 7
Full lips and stellate irises
Supravalvular aortic stenosis and peripheral pulmonary artery stenosis
Mild mental retardation
Check BP as increased risk of renal artery stenosis.

CAN YOU …

Talk through the examination features of aortic stenosis?
If shown an ECG what would you look for?
What features would you look for if told the cause of the aortic stenosis was related to a syndrome?

COMMENTS ON STATION 2

DIAGNOSIS: INFLAMMATORY BOWEL DISEASE

It is potentially possible to complete a large proportion of your SHO training with little experience of surgery and scars. Severe inflammatory bowel disease is generally treated by specialist gastroenterologists and surgeons and unless you have done a specific attachment your experience may be limited to the textbook. Knowledge of common surgical scars will either impress examiners or save embarrassment, depending on which way you look at it!

Nutritional assessment is commonly overlooked in revision. An entire short case may be devoted to it, so make sure you have an understanding of the principles involved.

Nutritional assessment	Notes
General	Weight/height/BMI Nasogastric placement Long-term venous access Does the patient look well?
Storage	Subcutaneous fat (mid-arm, subscapular and axillary) Muscle bulk (biceps, triceps and quadriceps) Prominence of iliac bones
Face	Pale conjunctiva Oral ulceration Dental caries
Skin	Liver disease and vitamin deficiency demonstrated by jaundice and bruising Rashes Excoriations Erythema nodosum
Hands	Pallor (of palmar creases) Clubbing of fingers Palmar erythema Koilonychia (dystrophy of the fingernails in which they are thinned and concave with raised edges; 'spoon-shaped nails') Leuconychia (white spots on the nails)
Abdomen	Distension Hepatosplenomegaly Surgical scars
Other	Gait examination: tests strength and any neurological impairment Blood pressure and pulse (standing and lying to measure postural change) Urinalysis and stool analysis as appropriate Pubertal assessment

Just because in books patients with Crohn's disease have aphthous ulcers (do you actually know what these are?), gum hyperplasia, little subcutaneous fat, anaemia, growth delay, peri-anal skin tags and signs of steroid toxicity doesn't mean your patient will.

[*Aphthous ulcer*: a shallow individual ulcer that is round or oval in shape. The ulcer will usually be no more than ¼ inch in diameter. The centre of the ulcer will be covered with a loosely attached white or greyish membrane. The edges of the ulcer will be regular (non-jagged) and surrounded by a reddish halo. The tissue adjacent to the ulcer will be healthy in appearance.]

Your growth-delayed, slightly pale teenager with a scar without signs of lymphoreticular disease (i.e. oncological) is likely to have an inflammatory bowel disease. If they have GI involvement outside of the colon, as evidenced by oral ulceration, then they are likely to have Crohn's but this is not absolute. What you must do is convince the examiner you are able to acknowledge growth delay or nutritional deficiency in a sensitive manner. You must then assess the most likely cause of this. Finally, be able to suggest some investigations and management both for the acute *and* non-acute situation.

Inflammatory bowel disease	Tips
Exam	Weight/height/BMI/head circumference Clubbing (rare) Cushingoid appearance or striae Scars from acute surgery (obstruction) or non-acute surgery (growth failure, debilitating symptoms, colectomy/pouch or prevention of malignancy), perineum, looking for anal fissures and skin tags
Investigations	*Blood tests:* (Leucocytosis, raised ESR, low protein, renal impairment, consider vitamins and minerals in long-term follow-up) *Stool:* Culture to exclude other diagnoses α_1-Antitrypsin (reflects bowel protein loss) *Imaging/endoscopy:* Left wrist X-ray for bone age AXR acutely Barium meal/follow-through dependent on position of lesion
Management: Crohn's	Multidisciplinary approach Use of steroids (orally or intravenous) Aware of sulfasalazine for small bowel disease May need steroid sparing agents: azathioprine, ciclosporin or methotrexate Nutritional therapies including use of overnight feeds
Management: ulcerative colitis	Multidisciplinary approach Steroid enemas or oral steroids Sulfasalazine for acute situation Yearly colonoscopy when disease >10–15 years

An example answer would be:

'I have examined John, who is a 15-year-old boy but appears underweight and small for his age. I would like to plot his height and weight on a growth chart. There appears to be peripheral muscle wasting and I need to assess this formally with skin-fold callipers and mid-arm circumference. He has pale conjunctivae but no obvious oral ulceration. There are no invasive feeding or intravenous lines. On abdominal examination there is a surgical scar consistent with a laparotomy but his abdomen is otherwise soft, with no masses. He has some diffuse tenderness at the left iliac fossa but no guarding. It would be useful to examine his peri-anal region for evidence of fissures or skin tags.

'This child may have an inflammatory bowel condition as evidenced by his stunted growth and previous abdominal surgery, which may have been necessary for a severe bout of colitis.'

REMINDER

A laparotomy scar will run transverse through the centre of the abdomen (see Fig. 4).

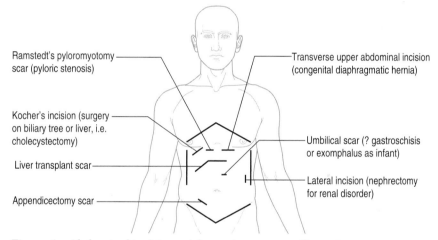

Figure 4   Abdominal incisions. A laparotomy scar will run transverse through the centre of the abdomen

CAN YOU …

Talk through your examination of a child's nutritional status with a colleague?

COMMENTS ON STATION 3

DIAGNOSIS: SYDENHAM'S CHOREA

The art of observation before examination is persistently stressed throughout your medical training. Although you may not have done this as a medical student it is essential you have the ability to 'hang back'. Engaging your brain before putting your mouth in gear will stop you blurting out an answer you will be unable to defend.

It is vital before the exam that you are able to talk about observed features in a systematic fashion. It is actually a very difficult thing to do; try talking about colleagues' gaits. Can you make an efficient summary without stopping, mumbling and being imprecise? The longer you are able to discuss things, the less time you have to be observed examining them – much the harder task!

Learning long lists of differentials is only helpful if you are able to pick up the signs that apply to them. In this situation you are expected to recognise chorea and possibly athetosis (with the appreciation that a written description is no substitute for actually having seen the clinical sign). The most obvious differential is a tic or habit spasm. These are repetitive and have a classical stereotypical pattern, but most importantly can be briefly controlled by the subject. The performance of the movement provides some brief relief.

It is useful to have a good understanding of the potential causes and apply those to the child in question. The examiner will expect you to be able to describe the irregular jerking movements and how the patient seems to have little control over them. They would then expect you to be able to mention additional signs (seen or unseen) that would aid a diagnosis, *not* just a list of differentials.

Compare: *'This child seems to have abnormal movements of their arms. They look like chorea to me. This may be as a result of cerebral palsy or Huntington's. I know Huntington's sometimes starts in childhood and has a very poor outlook.'*

To: *'This school-aged child is alert at rest. The most obvious feature is persistent involuntary movements of the limbs, particularly the arms. The arms show rapid movements in any direction and appear to cause the child distress. She has difficulty refraining from the movements. I also note occasional movements of the tongue and some facial twitching. Her head circumference looks normal for her age, although I will plot it on a growth chart and I need to do a thorough peripheral nervous system examination. In particular, I am looking at muscle strength and reflexes. I will examine the lower limbs, looking for evidence of spasticity. I am observing chorea which had multiple causes but in particular it may be part of the clinical picture of dyskinetic cerebral palsy.*
It is important I actively search for evidence of previous streptococcal infection as this may be a Sydenham's chorea. There are also a number of rarer metabolic or degenerative conditions for which a detailed family history must be taken.'

In the former you instantly lose the trust of the mother and the examiner wonders where you learned your bedside manner. The second demonstrates you are not just a walking textbook but able to apply your knowledge systematically and relevantly. This child had Sydenham's chorea.

Chorea	Notes
Anticonvulsant side effect	
Cerebral palsy – dyskinetic	Look specifically for athetosis (slow writhing movements) as cerebral palsy is the commonest cause of this Assess intellectual impairment, spastic posturing and gait
Sydenham's chorea	Acute-onset choreiform movements May have 'milkmaid's grip' – inconsistent hard and weak grasp of examining finger Extended hands tend to pronate Anaemia, leucocytosis and potential increased ESR Check ASO titre Throat swab for Group A haemolytic streptococci There may be a psychological element (emotional lability and depression) Treat with dopaminergic blockers (haloperidol) Remember this is a major manifestation of rheumatic fever and so is likely to need antistreptococcal rheumatic fever prophylaxis
Wilson's disease	Family history (autosomal recessive) Difficulty excreting copper in bile Low ceruloplasmin and increased urinary excretion of copper Evidence of liver failure (must examine abdomen of children with chorea) Copper chelate with D-penicillamine
Degenerative conditions (?appropriate for exam)	Huntington's disease, Lesch–Nyhan, Moyamoya

The following websites have video clips of choreiform movements and tics. The former is a superb revision aid, especially for developmental progression in the under-2-year-old (go to pediNeurologic exam):

library.med.utah.edu/neurologicexam/html/gait_abnormal.html
www.kcom.edu/faculty/chamberlain/Website/lectures/lecture/image/chorea.mov
www.issc.info/videoclipstourettempeg.html

The movements may be controlled by haloperidol, although it is important to discuss some of the important side effects and caveats with parents before commencing treatment. This would easily be the basis for a communication station.

1. Haloperidol can be useful in dampening down the involuntary spasms but unfortunately can actually make the movements worse.
2. The most important side effect is oculogyric crisis. This may cause the patient to have very forceful movements of their neck and head associated with rolling movements of the arms.
3. To prevent the above the dose of haloperidol must be initially small and increased slowly. If there are reactions, ceasing medication will prevent long-term problems.

Criteria for diagnosis of rheumatic fever (need two major or one major and two minor plus evidence of streptococcal disease)

Major	Plus
Carditis	Increased titres of antistreptolysin O
Polyarthritis	Positive throat culture for Group A streptococci
Sydenham's chorea	
Erythema marginatum	
Subcutaneous nodules	
(not erythema nodosum)	
Minor	After acute episode
Previous rheumatic fever	Need regular penicillin
Polyarthralgia	Follow-up of possible valvular damage
Fever	
Elevated CRP, ESR, WCC	
Prolonged P–R interval	

CAN YOU …

List the causes of chorea?
Describe which investigations you would perform on a child you suspect has Wilson's disease?

COMMENTS ON STATION 4

DIAGNOSIS: RIGHT BASAL PNEUMONIA

The new exam mark sheets have a specific box to assess whether the child is cooperative or not for the exam. As long as you have not provoked the child by doing something inappropriate or rough you cannot be penalised. In the stress of the exam it is easy to forget the 'child' and only remember the 'system'. Part of your introductory patter should involve some play with the child. Most importantly, get mother on your side! To some candidates this comes naturally but to others it may not be normal (or sometimes expected) for them to be involved in child's play. It is a skill as hard as picking up an atrial septal defect and probably should be practised as much!

Chronic respiratory disease is an easy provider of signs and symptoms so is well utilised in the exam. However, there is no reason that a previous acutely unwell child may be used. In this case there are specific features to elucidate, so have you been listening? Which side were the abnormal breath sounds on? Is there an inhaler/monitor/sputum pot by the bed? Do not stop listening until you are able to tell the examiner:

- what the child looks like at rest;
- whether the child is well grown;
- what items are around the bed;
- where the pathology is – make sure you are definite and have not confused right and left!
- what the pathology is – e.g., there is clubbing, not there may be clubbing.

This child is recovering from a right basal pneumonia but in order to make this diagnosis you must also know:

- the general health of the child when well;
- whether there is any evidence of chronic respiratory impairment;
- whether there is any evidence of immunodeficiency (must ask if child immunised);
- whether a CXR has been performed;
- whether a temperature reveals evidence of fever.

CAN YOU ...

List techniques you would use to entertain/distract a 4-year-old child?

COMMENTS ON STATION 5

DIAGNOSIS: FANCONI'S ANAEMIA

Having remembered long lists of odd syndromes and genetic variants for the previous two exams it would be nice to think there was something you could forget! Unfortunately, the 'other' station may bring up the odd curiosity despite the College's statement that this should be an exam of normal practice. Much like dermatological problems being linked to underlying neurological deficits, abnormalities of the arms, especially the radius and thumb, are linked to haematological disease. The two most common textbook examples are TAR (thrombocytopenia absent radius syndrome) and in this case Fanconi's anaemia. Sometimes you just have to know your stuff!

Fanconi's anaemia	Notes
Signs and symptoms	Anaemia causing weakness Neutropenia causing infections Thrombocytopenia causing bleeding and bruising Commonly have abnormal pigmentation of the skin May have short stature with skeletal malformations (absent thumb and radius – check it's there!) Renal anomalies
Laboratory findings	Macrocytic anaemia Thrombocytopenia precedes severe aplastic anaemia Rule out idiopathic thrombocytopenic purpura
Complications	Generally related to haematological dysfunction but there is also a significant risk of developing a malignancy, especially leukaemias and solid tumours

COMMENTS ON STATION 6

DIAGNOSIS: TREACHER COLLINS SYNDROME

Do you know your syndromes? For this case it actually doesn't matter, as you were asked to 'assess this child's speech and language'. In fact, it is very important not to get distracted by the obvious abnormalities. Even knowing the syndrome, if you cannot do a quick assessment of speech and hearing you will not be gaining the marks. Remember the College specifically say they are not testing you against the trained developmental paediatrician but the first-year registrar. Accepting this child is unlikely to present to an outpatient clinic at this age with concerns about speech and language, this must still be the approach to take.

Unless definitely told otherwise, it is appropriate to ask the mother about any concerns she has with regard to hearing and speech. The examiner may use this to ask further questions about how you would test specific deficits. Make sure you have seen audiological tests performed. You may well be asked to explain them in the communication skills station!

In the exam, as you do not have access to audiometry you must utilise simpler tests such as distraction testing. In fact, this simple test may be utilised for any age. While playing with the child (without noise), if you ask the examiner to call his name from behind him and he looks round every time then some element of hearing must be present (the converse is not true!). It can be difficult to show differences in each ear but the McCormick toy test may be used. Although used for a slightly younger age group (2–4 years) you do not have formal audiological testing to hand and neurological exam on the eighth cranial nerve is not an appropriate first step for this station. Pairs of similar sounding toys are placed in front of the child and the name of one whispered in each ear. It is important that the child cannot see your mouth as some children may have learnt basic lip-reading.

Listening to the child talk is vital as it is a functional sign of audiological ability. Poor quality or limited language for a 5-year-old in the absence of motor problems is likely to represent a degree of hearing impairment. Given the malformations, this may seem like an obvious diagnosis. The examiner is looking for how you approach the history and child.

Have you commented that the fine and gross motor skills appear normal? Is the child playing with toys that produce noise? How does he interact with his mother?

Note in the guidelines to the exam that the College specifically state that the child will have a developmental age of less than 5 years. This does *not* mean the child will be less than 5 years. It does mean that as long as you know development milestones up to 5 years of age you should at least be able to comment on whether the child is underachieving.

Causes of speech delay are listed below. Again, you are being assessed on your ability to recognise developmental abnormality, not to provide a list of differential diagnosis. This list should help you look for things to confirm your initial suspicions and maybe make comments on other features that support this – proving to the examiner you really are a well-rounded paediatrician!

	At 5 years
Gross motor	Stands on one foot for up to 10 seconds (and can therefore hop) Interest in climbing May be able to skip
Fine motor and vision	Copies triangle Draws person with body details Uses fork and spoon but not knife
Speech and hearing	Can count 10 objects Knows if morning or afternoon Can read words
Social	Knows name and address Can use large buttons in dressing and undressing Knows right and left hand Can do simple household tasks (helps with dishes)

CAUSES OF SPEECH DELAY

- Hearing loss
- Developmental language delay
- Bilingualism
- Social deprivation and/or neglect
- Cerebral palsy
- Elective mutism

This child had Treacher Collins syndrome with left-sided hearing loss but no other developmental delay.

TYPE OF HEARING TEST

- Distraction tests — 6–12 months
- Speech discrimination tests — 2–4 years
- Performance tests — 24–30 months
- Pure tone audiometry — 4–5 years
- Electrical response audiometry — Neonate
- Brain stem auditory evoked responses — Neonate
- Evoked otoacoustic emissions — Any age

REMINDER

Treacher Collins

- A syndrome characterised by maxillary hypoplasia and micrognathia
- Autosomal dominant
- Typical features
  - Down-slanting eyes
  - Sparse or absent eyelashes
  - Underdevelopment or absence of cheekbones and eye socket

– Small and slanting lower jaw
– Underdeveloped, malformed and/or prominent ears
- Sleep problems and/or sleep apnoea
- Benefit from early intervention of speech and language problems
- Intelligence usually normal.

COMMENTS ON STATION 7

The ability to communicate to professional colleagues is viewed as important as talking to parents. With the growing rise of Medical Education as a specialty in its own right, the ability to teach is increasingly seen as a prerequisite skill. In this scenario the important points are ensuring the student understands and can demonstrate the skill. Just running through BLS in front of the student may fail you if that is all you demonstrate. The student must be able to perform the tasks in the correct order without prompting. Obviously in 9 minutes it will be difficult to complete the task but an impression will be made of the rapport you make.

A proposed sequence is:

1. Introduce yourself and explain what you are going to do.
2. Ask for previous knowledge teaching.
3. Explain you are just doing basic airway management and help has been called for.
4. Ensure a *safe* approach.
5. Show airway technique (chin lift, jaw thrust).
6. Assess breathing (look, listen, feel).
7. Five rescue breaths if no breathing.
8. Assess circulation (brachial or femoral). Commence chest compression if no pulse or pulse less than 60.
9. Show cardiac compression (heel of one hand over the lower third of the sternum, one finger breadth above the xiphisternum).
10. Commence CPR at 15:2 ratio until help arrives. Compression rate 100 per minute.

Just reading these pointers will be of little help. It is vital you are observed performing this exercise with a colleague by a senior paediatrician who can give you feedback. It is amazing how quickly a simple task becomes complex when you are observed doing it!

At each point the student should demonstrate their understanding and be able to do the practical task. If you have time you may demonstrate the whole scenario to them and get them to do the same.

Make sure you are familiar with the latest Advanced Paediatric Life Support Guidelines.

COMMENTS ON STATION 8

Although this may seem like an unlikely scenario and not particularly the duty of a first-year registrar, there are many times when family members have certain questions which are appropriate for you to answer. The brain stem death test is not something which will be carried out by a registrar but is something with which you should at least be aware. The essence of this case is how you approach the very sensitive issue of death. The principles of good preparation are vital. You must introduce yourself with full name and position. Tell Mark you have diverted your pager and ask if he would like anyone else present. It may be worthwhile suggesting a nurse accompany you.

An initial statement saying how sorry you are for the situation is essential. The sequence of questions/answers from here is difficult to predict and it would seem sensible to take your lead from Mark. It may be that Mark may show signs of distress or even anger at the care his sister has received. This is an understandable reaction and can be addressed as such. Remember actors may be employed and will demonstrate accurate and very real representations of people's emotions. Ultimately the overall issue is that Stephanie has died and the machines are providing complete life support for her. It would be inappropriate, in order to deflect some of Mark's anger, to suggest there may be a positive outcome. The brain stem death test is a legal requirement and is used to confirm but not diagnose, i.e. don't say 'Well, let's wait to see what the test shows'. There may be a certain amount of guilt that he was not around and he may blame members of staff or his family. You will be marked on your ability to listen as well as explain and you may have to repeatedly stress that you understand this is a difficult time for him. Make sure that at completion you check you have answered Mark's questions and that if he has any more at any time he should contact a member of staff.

Mark is likely to want to know what the test involves (see below) and who will be carrying it out.

Clinical brain stem death exam

Establish cause of disease/injury and:	
Coexistence of coma and apnoea	Apnoea test; observe for 3 minutes with $PCO_2 > 60$ mmHg
Absence of brain stem function	Fully dilated pupils with no light response Absence of spontaneous eye movement and those produced by doll's eye movements and water instillation in external auditory meatus Corneal and gag reflexes absent
Normal blood pressure and temperature	
Flaccid muscle tone, no spontaneous movement	
Exam consistent through observation period	Two exams over 12–24 hours

COMMENTS ON STATION 9

In may be argued that specialist diabetic management does not fall within the remit of the first-year specialist registrar. However, diabetes is a common disease and is managed by district general hospitals. Knowledge of the disease is required and, in particular, dealing with the 'difficult' teenager is an art form in itself. It must be emphasised that this is outpatient management. A diatribe on acute symptoms is not going to help you pass the station. The scenario revolves around a previously well-controlled child (knowledge of HbA1c levels is assumed) who now has poor control.

You must be aware of and take a thorough history of all aspects of the way diabetes affects children. This involves:

History	Notes
Initial diagnosis	Age Intervention needed (?PICU) Length of hospital stay Education given
Past management history	Number of hospitalisations (including PICU) Frequency of monitoring Changes of management Complications of treatment (lipohypertrophy, hypoglycaemic episodes)
Current treatment	Type of insulin and duration of this treatment Modifications for sport, etc. Frequency of monitoring Dietary adaptations (is there a dietician involved?)
Social history	*Effects on child:* Understanding of disease and long-term complications *Effects on friends and school:* Any involvement in diabetic camps/groups? *Effect on family:* Siblings' understanding of disease Involvement of social worker Change of family's diet

The key to the management plan is being able to ascertain what the change has been and coming up with an *appropriate* way of addressing this issue. It may be that a change in insulin prescription has not been correctly followed up. Advising a diabetic nurse review of the doses/glucose monitoring while awaiting specialist follow-up may simply be the answer. However, it is more likely there are a number of issues pertaining to Steven's adolescence. Monitoring may well be less rigid than previously and at this stage in Steven's life a night spent drinking has much more short-term gain than long-term good glucose control! It is important to give encouragement rather than chastisement. Management of psychological issues must make use of the whole family and may involve support groups or individual counselling in some cases. Diabetic nurses/social workers are an essential resource but should not be assumed to be involved.

REMINDER

Examination must include:

- Height and weight
- Fundoscopy
- Blood pressure (hypertension)
- Urinalysis (presence of urinalysis)
- Injection sites.

Rapid, short- and long-acting insulins are all available to enable:

- Twice daily (short- and long-acting)
- Basal bolus (rapid before meals and long-acting overnight)
- Twice daily, basal bolus combinations
- Continuous infusions.

General requirement 0.7–1.0 Units/day, increasing to 1.0–1.5 Units/day with the pubertal growth spurt.

Circuit D

STATION 1

This station assesses your ability to elicit clinical signs:
- **CVS**

This is a 9-minute station of clinical interaction. You will have up to 4 minutes beforehand to prepare yourself. No additional information will be given or is necessary before commencing the station. When the bell sounds you will be invited into the examination room.

INTRODUCTION

On entering the station you are presented with a boy approximately 8 years old. You are told, 'Please examine Jonathan's cardiovascular system and present your findings'.

CLINICAL SCENARIO

The child looks well. Peripheral examination is normal. The only positive examination findings are an obvious thrill at the lower left sternal edge and a harsh systolic murmur heard throughout the precordium but loudest at the lower left sternal edge.

What do you say to the examiner?

This station assesses your ability to elicit clinical signs:

- Abdo/Other

This is a 9-minute station of clinical interaction. You will have up to 4 minutes beforehand to prepare yourself. No additional information will be given or is necessary before commencing the station. When the bell sounds you will be invited into the examination room.

INTRODUCTION

On entering the station you are presented with a girl approximately 4 years old. You are told, 'Please examine Sally's abdominal system and then present your findings'.

CLINICAL SCENARIO

The Caucasian child looks well. She is not obviously anaemic and you cannot convince yourself whether she is jaundiced or not. Her abdomen is soft and non-tender. Her spleen is palpable to three finger-breadths and you cannot feel a liver. There is no other obvious clinical sign present.

What do you say to the examiner?

Why does her mother have a scar in her right hypochondrium?

STATION 3

This station assesses your ability to elicit clinical signs:
- **Neurological**

This is a 9-minute station of clinical interaction. You will have up to 4 minutes beforehand to prepare yourself. No additional information will be given or is necessary before commencing the station. When the bell sounds you will be invited into the examination room.

INTRODUCTION

On entering the station you are presented with a 2- to 3-year-old girl. She is obviously microcephalic and developmentally delayed. The examiner invites you to comment on her appearance.

CLINICAL SCENARIO

You note her microcephaly and comment that her gaze seems deconjugate. The child is then asked to walk across the room and back. At this point you notice she is wearing ankle supports (ankle–foot orthoses: AFOs). Both her hips and knees are flexed and the weight of her body seems to be balanced on her toes. In order to move forwards she rotates her body to one side to bring forward her leading foot. The examiner asks you what you would like to examine next.

What do you say and what will you be looking for?

This station assesses your ability to elicit clinical signs:

- **Respiratory/Other**

This is a 9-minute station of clinical interaction. You will have up to 4 minutes beforehand to prepare yourself. No additional information will be given or is necessary before commencing the station. When the bell sounds you will be invited into the examination room.

INTRODUCTION

On entering the room you are presented with a boy approximately 12 years old who is sitting upright on a couch without his top on. There is a semicircular scar above the left nipple. He breathes easily with a normal respiratory rate. You are asked to examine his respiratory system.

CLINICAL SCENARIO

Clinical examination is unremarkable although you are unsure as to whether he is hyperexpanded or not. You mention this to the examiner, who asks you how you would confirm this.

He then tells you the child has been suffering from persistent chest infections for some time now.

What must you examine his hands for?

What investigations would you like to do?

STATION 5

This station assesses your ability to elicit clinical signs:

- **Other**

This is a 9-minute station of clinical interaction. You will have up to 4 minutes beforehand to prepare yourself. No additional information will be given or is necessary before commencing the station. When the bell sounds you will be invited into the examination room.

INTRODUCTION

On entering the room you are presented with an adolescent girl. She looks well. The examiner informs you she has had multiple falls recently and her mother is worried she has become clumsy when she walks. Please assess this child.

How will you commence your examination?

CLINICAL SCENARIO

You examine her gait and it is entirely normal. You can find no problems with her balance and her lower limbs have normal tone, power and reflexes. You are perplexed until you notice that her left leg appears larger than her right.

How will you proceed?

This station assesses your ability to assess specifically requested areas in a child with a developmental problem:

• **Development**

This is a 9-minute station of clinical interaction. You will have up to 4 minutes beforehand to prepare yourself. No additional information will be given or is necessary before commencing the station. When the bell sounds you will be invited into the examination room.

INTRODUCTION

You are informed that the child you are to assess is 3 years old. You are asked to examine her speech and language development.

How do you proceed?

CLINICAL SCENARIO

Her mother tells you that she only uses two to three words maximum and apart from 'no' the other words are unrecognisable.

The examiner would like you to demonstrate that she truly understands specific tasks requested of her.

This station assesses your ability to communicate appropriate, factually correct information in an effective way within the emotional context of the clinical setting:

- **Communication One**

This is a 9-minute station consisting of spoken interaction. You will have up to 2 minutes before the start of the station to read this sheet and prepare yourself. You may make notes on the paper provided.

When the bell sounds you will be invited into the examination room. Please take this instruction sheet with you. The examiner will not ask questions during the 9 minutes but will warn you when you have approximately 2 minutes left.

You are not required to examine a patient.

The encounter should be focused on the task; you will be penalised for asking irrelevant questions or providing superfluous information. You will be marked on your ability to communicate, not the speed with which you convey information. You may not have time to complete the communication.

SETTING

You are a specialist registrar in paediatrics working in a district hospital.

SCENARIO

Your SHO has seen a 6-month-old child whom you suspect may have meningitis. You wish to perform a lumbar puncture before commencing antibiotics. Please explain this procedure to the child's mother. She is aware of why the lumbar puncture must take place and you need *not* take any further history.

This station assesses your ability to communicate appropriate, factually correct information in an effective way within the emotional context of the clinical setting:

- **Communication Two**

This is a 9-minute station consisting of spoken interaction. You will have up to 2 minutes before the start of the station to read this sheet and prepare yourself. You may make notes on the paper provided.

When the bell sounds you will be invited into the examination room. Please take this instruction sheet with you. The examiner will not ask questions during the 9 minutes but will warn you when you have approximately 2 minutes left.

You are not required to examine a patient.

The encounter should be focused on the task; you will be penalised for asking irrelevant questions or providing superfluous information. You will be marked on your ability to communicate, not the speed with which you convey information. You may not have time to complete the communication.

SETTING

You are a neonatal registrar for a tertiary neonatal unit.

SCENARIO

You have just completed a neonatal ward round. You spent some time discussing Robert, an ex-24-week preterm infant who is now 27 weeks corrected. He has had a stormy course and is still ventilated. However, his respiratory condition is improving and it is hoped he will be put onto CPAP soon. He has recently started feeds, having been on a course of TPN. He has avoided any septic complications but unfortunately has biventricular grade 4 haemorrhages on ultrasound scan. A medical student, Tanya, asks why the team are still treating Robert, as she has heard this kind of haemorrhage always leads to cerebral palsy and isn't this unfair?

Tanya is on an attachment to the unit and is well known to you. A prolonged introduction is unnecessary. She is also familiar with Robert's history so you need only focus on the relevant issues to answer her question.

STATION 9

This station assesses your ability to take a focused history and explain to the parent your diagnosis or differential management plan:

- History-taking and Management planning

This is a 22-minute station of spoken interaction. You will have up to 4 minutes beforehand to prepare yourself. The scenario is below. Be aware that you should focus on the task given. You will be penalised for asking irrelevant questions or providing superfluous information. When the bell sounds you will be invited into the examination room. You will have 13 minutes with the patient (with a warning when you have 4 minutes left). You will then have a short period to reflect on the case while the patient leaves the room. You will then have 9 minutes with the examiner.

INFORMATION

You are a paediatric SpR working in a general outpatient clinic in a district general hospital, where you have received the following letter:

Dear Doctor

Re: Monique 7 years

Thank you for seeing Monique, whose family have recently returned from France, where they have been living for the past 7 years. Monique's mother is English and tells me she has been diagnosed with cystic fibrosis. She was managed by a medical team in France but a transfer letter they had written has been lost. Her mother has kindly listed some of the medications she is on but I am not familiar with all of them. I feel Monique needs some more specialist management and was hoping you could make a detailed referral to the closest tertiary centre.

Your help is appreciated.

PS. Monique is on the 2nd centile for weight and 9th for height.

Take a history from Monique and her mother, for whom you have no background history. Discuss your referral and management plan with the examiner. You do not need to explain your plan to Monique's mother.

DIAGNOSIS: VENTRICULOSEPTAL DEFECT

'I have examined Jonathan, who is a well-looking boy, and I would like to plot his height and weight on a growth chart. There is no evidence of cardiorespiratory distress and positive findings are a thrill at the left sternal edge with a grade 4 pansystolic murmur loudest in this region. This is a VSD and I note there is no evidence of heart failure.'

With ventriculoseptal defects being the most common congenital cardiac anomaly, these (one would hope) will be the murmurs you are likely to hear. The VSD is a must-know station. You must be able to diagnose this with confidence. For some candidates this will mean hunting high and low for a cardiology clinic or attending a specific course. The advantage of assured diagnosis is not only in the confidence it will give you in the exam but also the examiner will find it much easier to test you. Easy marks are subsequently gained for knowing investigations, antibiotic prophylaxis and indications for surgery. These cannot be asked if you are still deliberating as to whether it is aortic stenosis!

	Tips
Exam	A loud second heart sound suggests pulmonary hypertension (from a large shunt) until proven otherwise Feel the suprasternal notch (a thrill there means AS, or rarely PS) A thrill means the murmur must be grade 4: **1** Soft and heard with difficulty **2** Soft but easily heard **3** Loud but without thrill **4** Loud and associated with thrill **5** Loud, with thrill but stethoscope must be in contact with chest wall **6** Audible without the use of a stethoscope
Investigations	ECG and CXR (can be done at any hospital so a better first-line investigation) – normal if insignificant/asymptomatic *Signs of heart failure:* – Cardiomegaly – Diastolic murmur at apex – LVH on ECG ECHO – 2D
Diagnosis	An asymptomatic murmur suggestive of VSD may be monitored clinically (the confident paediatrician may not even do an ECHO; not wise to suggest in exam if you are not sure!)
Management	Control congestive cardiac failure (diuretics/captopril) Maintain normal growth with calorie supplementation Surgery if pulmonary to systemic flow ratio > 2:1 Good dental hygiene with antibiotic prophylaxis (amoxicillin) for procedures

REMINDER

All Down's syndrome children should be routinely sent for an echo-cardiogram (VSD, AVSD). These children are at high risk of developing pulmonary hypertension and subsequently Eisenmenger's complex with large shunts.

Heart failure

Neonatal	Infancy	Any
Hypoplastic left heart	VSD	SVT
Aortic coarctation	AVSD	Myocarditis
Aortic stenosis	PDA (large)	Cardiomyopathy
Tricuspid atresia	TAPVD	
Interrupted aortic arch		

DID YOU ...

Ask for a blood pressure?
Feel the femoral pulses?
Feel for hepatomegaly?
Listen to the back of the chest?
Plot the patient's height and weight?

COMMENTS ON STATION 2

DIAGNOSIS: HEREDITARY SPHEROCYTOSIS

'I have examined Sally, who looks well, and I would like to plot her height and weight. My positive findings are a spleen measuring three finger-breadths below the left costal margin. Although she does not look anaemic and her sclera do not look overtly jaundiced, the most likely cause for her splenomegaly is hereditary spherocytosis. I would like to take a history and rule out the presence of a myeloproliferative disorder or infection before establishing this diagnosis.'

Contrary to popular belief in the hot, stuffy and brightly lit exam room, it is not always easy to pick up peripheral signs of abdominal disease. When one of the authors mentioned he was unable to detect evidence of anaemia in his patient, her mother immediately said, 'I know, I have never seen her cheeks look so rosy!'. The examiner admitted the patient looked neither jaundiced nor anaemic despite the diagnosis and the candidate was spared the blushes of admitting he had made up signs he thought should have been there.

Hereditary spherocytosis	Tips
Exam	Cholecystectomy scar (more likely the older the patient) and a splenectomy scar
Treatment	Remember folic acid supplements Pneumococcal, meningococcal and *Haemophilus influenzae* B immunisation required Lifelong penicillin prophylaxis
Acute management	Aplastic crises can occur Pigmented gallstones present in majority by second decade
Differentials	Hereditary elliptocytosis Autoimmune haemolytic anaemia

The mother has had her gallstones removed (also having hereditary spherocytosis!).

CAN YOU …

Explain a new diagnosis of hereditary spherocytosis to a family who are unfamiliar with the condition?

COMMENTS ON STATION 3

DIAGNOSIS: CEREBRAL PALSY

There is no excuse for not knowing your neurological exam inside out. The difficulty for some candidates is that, despite knowing how to perform the 'perfect' exam, the application and interpretation of the results are still difficult. You are also faced with the problem of guessing what the examiner would like you to do. It is very easy to get distracted from your examination routine because you are concerned about getting the whole answer.

For example, the candidate in our scenario notices the microcephaly and wants to examine the patient's eyes. The examiner, having demonstrated a spastic gait, is annoyed as he feels he has given a clue to examine the lower limbs. He informs the candidate of this, so they go on to look at the legs. While examining the lower limbs, the examiner then becomes annoyed by the thoroughness of the candidate. Having demonstrated a microcephalic child with a spastic gait he feels you should quickly demonstrate just the increased tone and brisk reflexes. He says, 'If you're not quick you won't have time to look at the eyes' – which the candidate was stopped from doing in the first place!

It is probably easier to examine peripherally rather than centrally when you are under pressure. Therefore examine the legs first, giving yourself time to collect your thoughts. Don't be distracted by neurological signs in isolation, i.e. the eye signs must be taken with the microcephaly and spasticity.

As your head doesn't tend to shrink, it is likely an insult has occurred early in life.

In the neurological exam you must always be thinking:

What am I seeing? A neurologically disadvantaged child with multiple handicaps.

Why am I examining this limb? Spastic gait indicates upper motor neurone lesion.

What am I looking for? Increased tone and reflexes with clonus. Reduced power.

What am I finding? Is there wasting? Are the abnormalities symmetrical?

Learn a good definition of cerebral palsy and know some causes (although in this case you can only give a differential).

> *'Cerebral palsy is a persistent but variable disorder of movement and posture due to a non-progressive disorder of the developing brain.'*

Prenatal	Genetic TORCH IUGR Maternal alcohol/substance misuse
Perinatal	Hypoxic ischaemic encephalopathy Ventricular haemorrhage Hypoglycaemia
Postnatal	Meningitis/encephalitis Head injury

REMINDER

A *functional* assessment should reveal what a child *can* do. Therefore if asked to perform this specific instruction, in the appropriately aged child, ask:

'Can you show me how you would comb your hair?'
'Can you hold this knife and fork?'
'Can you sit up without using your hands?'
'Can you drink from this cup?'
'Can you show me how you put your shirt on in the morning?'

A quick way to uncover/ascertain a multidisciplinary approach is via the 'POSH' questionnaire:

P Physiotherapy involvement
O Occupational therapy involvement
S School/education involvement
H Home circumstances (social work involvement)

DIAGNOSIS: PREVIOUS PNEUMONIA LEADING TO BRONCHIECTASIS (UNABLE TO DETERMINE THIS FROM INFORMATION GIVEN)

A frustrating element of the exam is sometimes there not being an 'answer'. Many children are diagnostic dilemmas and have had multiple investigations, many treatments and thousands of membership candidates prodding and poking them. It is easy to convince yourself a sign *must* be there. To misquote the Jedi Master Yoda: *'Maybe not. A clinical sign or no clinical sign. There is no maybe.'*

Producing a list of possible investigations is of no benefit if you don't know *why* you are doing that test.

The differential diagnosis of chronic cough amongst all ages:

- Asthma — History and exam
- Congestive cardiac failure — History and exam
- H-type tracheo-oesophageal fistula — Radio-imaging
- Vascular ring — Radio-imaging
- Gastro-oesophageal reflux — History/pH study
- Lymphadenopathy — Exam
  - TB — Mantoux/CXR
  - Hodgkinson's — Biopsy/FBC
- Foreign body — History and radio-imaging
- Immunodeficiency states Functional antibodies — Immunoglobulins
- CF — Sweat test
- α_1-Antitrypsin deficiency — Protease inhibitor typing

Exam	Scars on the chest may be from surgical lines (?for antibiotics)
	Hyperexpansion:
	Without clubbing – asthma or chronic lung disease
	With clubbing – cystic fibrosis or bronchiectasis
	Other – persistent aspiration, tracheo-oesophageal fistula
	Hyperexpansion may be diagnosed clinically (increased AP diameter or displaced liver) or radiologically

It is vital in the respiratory case that an effort is made to assess the presence of clubbing, as you can see from the above table that the differential diagnosis is radically changed.

This child was not clubbed and his chest wall was not overtly hyperexpanded. You are told the cystic fibrosis screen was negative. Further history reveals he had a severe pneumonia a couple of years ago which has left him with permanent lung damage and some evidence of evolving bronchiectasis. Repeated chest infections have been a problem and while you were examining his hands you note a paucity of veins for his age (explaining the need for definitive access).

Causes of clubbing	Clubbing is not seen before 6 months of age
Cardiac	Congenital cyanotic heart disease Subacute bacterial endocarditis
Respiratory	Bronchiectasis/cystic fibrosis Primary ciliary dyskinesia Tuberculosis Empyema Malignancy Fibrosis
GI	Inflammatory bowel disease Biliary cirrhosis

COMMENTS ON STATION 5

DIAGNOSIS: NEUROFIBROMATOSIS

Unlike Station 4, when the answer might not be obtainable from the examination findings alone, it may be just you who doesn't have a clue! In this scenario the candidate recognised the large right leg and remembered something about hemihypertrophy and renal masses (suggesting an ultrasound when asked about investigations). He was asked what else he would examine and drew a blank. The examiner then demonstrated the large ipsilateral arm and an even more obvious unilateral tongue enlargement. The candidate had no idea and left deflated and confused, only noticing the *café au lait* spots as he left the room. Subsequently he passed the station probably just for picking up the original sign. Until you get the mark sheet you do not know how you have performed!

Hemihypertrophy	May involve whole side of body or just one limb May be congenital Associated with Wilms' tumours Occurs in Beckwith–Wiedemann syndrome Russell–Silver syndrome
Regional overgrowth	Neurofibromatosis type 1 (see summary on p.190) Haemangiomas

REMINDER

Russell–Silver dwarfism

This condition almost invariably has prenatal onset with IUGR. There is no specific gene known to cause the disease.

Should have	Commonly have	May have
Growth failure	Infant hypocalcaemia	*Café au lait spots*
Triangular shaped facies	Hemihypertrophy	Learning difficulty
Poor feeding in infancy	Micrognathia	
Clinodactyly (fifth finger)		

McCune–Albright syndrome (Albright's syndrome)

- Also known as polyostotic fibrous dysplasia
- Premature puberty
- Abnormal fibrous development of bone
- *Café au lait* spots.

It is *not* Albright's hereditary osteodystrophy, which is type 1 pseudohypoparathyroidism (no phosphaturic response to PTH) and has the following features:

- Short stature
- Obesity
- Shortening of fourth and fifth metacarpals
- Mild learning difficulties.

CAN YOU ...

List causes of *café au lait* spots?

- Ataxia telangiectasia:
  - Spinocerebellar degeneration
  - Low IgA and eosinophilia
  - Thymic hypoplasia (increased infections)
- Tuberous sclerosis
- Fanconi's anaemia
- McCune–Albright syndrome
- Russell–Silver dwarfism
- Bloom's syndrome:
  - Autosomal recessive (and exceedingly rare)
  - Growth delay
  - High rate of malignancies
- Gaucher's disease:
  - Lysosomal storage condition
  - Hepatosplenomegaly
- Chédiak–Higashi syndrome:
  - Blonde hair
  - Neutrophil phagocyte defect
  - Thrombocytopenia
  - Decreased intelligence
- Normal child!

COMMENTS ON STATION 6

DIAGNOSIS: ISOLATED SPEECH DELAY

Candidates commonly forget that specific elements will be asked for. In this case only speech and language are being assessed, so the child *copying* a circle will not gain you marks. However, if told to *draw* a circle this shows a certain level of language appreciation and at least the ability to hear. But if the child is barely three (may not be able to draw a circle) then this is an unfair request. Therefore you need not only to know your developmental milestones inside out, but you must also be precise about the area they are testing and know how to apply them consistently.

Unless directed otherwise, it is entirely reasonable to ask the mother her child's level of functioning. *'Can your child hear and see?'* will save 9 minutes of embarrassment.

Asking the child to place certain objects inside a cup or take them out of a box assesses understanding and requires only a small level of gross motor functioning.

If you have a visual memory the College-recommended *Child Development: An Illustrated Guide* is very useful.

REMINDER

The McCormick Speech Discrimination Test uses 14 paired words which should be recognisable by children from the age of approximately 2 years old. A set of toys are placed in front of the child, and the child is asked to name them all (the toy is removed if not identified correctly). The examiner covers his mouth and asks the child to show him or her one of the toys. The ideal level is 40 dB but in the exam situation you are merely demonstrating the principle.

Examples

Tree	Key
Man	Lamb
Plane	Plate
Cup	Duck

COMMENTS ON STATION 7

Explanation of a lumbar puncture must be something the candidate has encountered and performed on a number of occasions. There is no best way to do it but it is easy to do it badly and lose easily gained marks. You are being marked on your communication and empathic skills, *not* your history-taking and management. Therefore don't get bogged down in whys and wherefores. Asking a mother about the child's current state of health will instantly lose you marks. If you find it difficult to jump straight into things then make up some background banter; for example:

'I gather it has previously been explained to you why we need to perform a lumbar puncture, is that right? ... Good. We have performed some blood tests

to look for infection and make sure there will not be a risk of bleeding during the procedure. A lumbar puncture is ...'

A generalised answer should include the following:

1. Introduction (name and position); explain you will not be bleeped.
2. Confirmation of mother's relation to child and understanding of situation.
3. Does she want a relative or friend with her?
4. Explanation of the need to find a cause for the child's illness and what a septic screen involves.
5. Specific details of a lumbar puncture.
6. Allay fears regarding neurological damage and pain.
7. Specifically state the need to hold the child securely (stating this is usually the most uncomfortable part for the child).
8. Ability to give antibiotics regardless of success of procedure.

Ensure the mother understands all you have said.

COMMENTS ON STATION 8

Explaining to a medical student the ethics of withdrawing care is a mammoth task. Healthcare professional interaction is going to become an increasingly prominent part of the communication skills section and should not be off-putting for the candidate. Nine minutes is not really long enough to cover all the salient points, but remember that the instructions implicitly state you need not cover everything. Unless you have interacted with medical students over this issue before it is also difficult to know how to approach this issue. Do you give them a didactic talk or ask them questions on what they know? One author has passed a station using the asking-questions approach, so the College obviously are flexible in their approach.

Ethics will be a vital component to at least one of the communication skills stations. For this scenario, knowledge of the RCPCH guidelines on withdrawing care is essential. There are five situations in which withholding or withdrawing care is acceptable:

1. *The brain dead child*: A determination of brain stem death made by accepted medical standards.
2. *The permanent vegetative state*: 'A state of unawareness of self and environment in which the patient breathes spontaneously, has a stable circulation and shows cycles of eye closure and eye opening which simulate sleep and waking, for a period of 12 months following a head injury or 6 months following other causes of brain damage.'
3. *The no-hope/chance situation*: Treatment will delay death but will do nothing to improve the quality of life; there is no potential.
4. *The 'no-purpose' situation*: Continued treatment will not affect prognosis and may in fact make things worse. Things are likely to deteriorate with time.
5. *The unbearable situation*: Continued treatment and its effects are more than the family and/or child accepts, although it may be of some benefit.

How these are discussed or brought up is difficult and, I think, to the candidate's advantage. Demonstration or awareness of principles will be the important factors. Prowess at teaching, as everyone is aware, is not proportional to the intelligence of the teacher!

A suggested strategy is as follows:

1. Introduce yourself.
2. Assess understanding of ventricular haemorrhages in neonates.

Grade	Description	Mortality/disability
1	Isolated germinal matrix haemorrhage	6%/18%
2	Intraventricular haemorrhage with normal ventricle size	33%/36%
3	Intraventricular haemorrhage of sufficient severity to dilate ventricles with blood	60%/75%
4	Intraparenchymal haemorrhage	93%/75%

Parenchmal haemorrhage will resolve or develop into periventricular leucomalacia or a porencephalic cyst. Perventricular leucomalacia has a poor prognosis in terms of neurodevelopmental outcome.

3. Does she understand the four principles of ethics (autonomy, non-maleficence, beneficence and justice)?
4. At this stage does Robert fulfil any of the criteria for withdrawing care (open to interpretation – remember you are discussing the principles; there is no right or wrong answer). Ultimately we have no way of knowing Robert's level of functioning at this point and what his degree of neurological compromise will be.
5. Discuss that withdrawing care is a group decision that must involve the parents and multiple members of the healthcare team.

COMMENTS ON STATION 9

An offshoot of the long case but designed to be more representative of clinical practice, the history and management planning station is easy to overlook in revision. Interestingly, because you have two communication skills stations, the station should really only focus on the history taken from parents. As stated in the Introduction, it is difficult not to get tied up in explanation/communication to the parents during your history-taking. It will be important to avoid doing this, especially in this example, as you will have so little time to cover all the necessary ground.

For the station in question the salient points are the ability to differentiate between issues which are important for the GP, i.e. regular medications, stability of condition and emergency treatment, as opposed to those which should be referred to a tertiary centre, such as treatment modalities. Tertiary centre referral is the essence of your management plan but not the answer. What the question is looking for is whether you have enough experience of chronic disease to enable you to start a pathway that provides for the complete needs of the patient:

1. A brief but thorough background of Monique's past (how diagnosed, genetic analysis, disease progression in the first years of life).
2. Previous hospitalisations – acute or booked.
3. Respiratory status (lung function, microbiological colonisation, especially ABPA (allergic bronchopulmonary aspergillosis), current antibiotic regimens, DNase, treatment of coexisting asthma, physiotherapy).
4. Gastrointestinal disease (past and present complications, especially meconium ileus equivalent but also including rectal prolapse, growth, dietary and pancreatic supplements, dietician involvement, diabetic progression).
5. Social situation and family support.
6. Immunisations (influenza, pertussis and measles – easily forgotten!).

Nutritional status is vital and easily overlooked, as is the effect of the condition on the family. All these factors are difficult to elucidate in 13 minutes, and in the preparation period it may be worth noting information you need that the GP must be told. There is no harm at the end of the consultation saying, *'I think we should schedule another appointment to discuss some areas we haven't covered today'.*

NUTRITIONAL HINTS

1. Have you plotted figures on a growth chart (or at the very least asked to)?
2. Have you got serial measurements or a parent record of growth across time?
3. Do you understand the mechanisms of malnutrition?
   - Malabsorption increasing losses.
   - Increased energy needs (recurrent infection/inflammation or work of breathing, etc.).
   - Reduced intake (recurrent vomiting/diarrhoea or anorexia).
4. Does the child have supplements to aid malabsorption (pancreatic in CF)?
5. Is a dietician involved?
6. How do the family adjust their diet to help the child?

Already you can see that there is a massive amount to cover in the 13 minutes available. The examiner will be looking for the candidate who is able to cover a large amount of ground quickly but without rushing. They will need to highlight points which require immediate input, at the same time elucidating factors which will need long-term management. Experience in CF (and other chronic disease) clinics will be invaluable in getting an overview of the complex needs of these patients. As stated previously, you must be observed by senior staff taking histories as it is something you will have rarely done since being a student.

Circuit E

STATION 1

This station assesses your ability to elicit clinical signs:
- CVS

INTRODUCTION

You are asked to examine a 9-month-old baby's cardiovascular system.

CLINICAL SCENARIO

The baby is well grown and does not look dysmorphic. There is no peripheral cyanosis or stigmata of cardiovascular disease. You cannot see any scars or feel any thrills. On auscultation you note an ejection systolic murmur in the pulmonary area and an ejection click.

What have you examined to conclude there are no stigmata of cardiovascular disease?

What are your conclusions?

In what conditions might you see this abnormality?

STATION 2

This station assesses your ability to elicit clinical signs:

• **Abdo/Other**

This is a 9-minute station of clinical interaction. You will have up to 4 minutes beforehand to prepare yourself. No additional information will be given or is necessary before commencing the station. When the bell sounds you will be invited into the examination room.

INTRODUCTION

You are asked to examine the abdominal system of a 15-year-old boy.

CLINICAL SCENARIO

On inspection you note he is short for his age. He is sitting bare-chested on an inclined bench. He lacks muscle bulk and has no chest or axillary hair. You note a thoracolumbar kyphosis and bilateral hearing aids. He has a prominent forehead, large tongue and pronounced lips.

On assessing the abdominal system you note the positive findings of hepato-splenomegaly and a scar in the left inguinal region.

Can you bring these findings together in one diagnosis?

His eye examination is normal.

How would you stage his pubertal level?

STATION 3

This station assesses your ability to elicit clinical signs:

- **Neurological**

This is a 9-minute station of clinical interaction. You will have up to 4 minutes beforehand to prepare yourself. No additional information will be given or is necessary before commencing the station. When the bell sounds you will be invited into the examination room.

INTRODUCTION

You are asked to comment on and examine as appropriate a 9-month-old baby boy who is with his mother.

CLINICAL SCENARIO

You immediately notice a protuberance over the left side of his skull and a pipe-like structure crossing the triangles of his neck, with a small scar in the left upper quadrant of his abdomen. His head appears slightly larger than normal for his body size. You note that he has horizontal nystagmus with a convergent left squint.

As he is happily playing with a toy you are using to entertain him, you note he does not move his left arm or leg. He has generally increased tone on his left side with decreased power and brisk reflexes.

What are your conclusions?

How would you offer to investigate this child further?

This station assesses your ability to elicit clinical signs:
- **Respiratory/Other**

This is a 9-minute station of clinical interaction. You will have up to 4 minutes beforehand to prepare yourself. No additional information will be given or is necessary before commencing the station. When the bell sounds you will be invited into the examination room.

INTRODUCTION

On entering the station you are asked to examine a 12-year-old girl who has recently moved to the UK from India. She has been referred to you because she has suffered from a chronic cough for several years. The GP has found that a series of antibiotics and a course of oral steroids have been unhelpful.

CLINICAL SCENARIO

The girl of Asian origin is very shy and quiet. On examination you notice early clubbing, a hyperexpanded chest, Harrison sulci and coarse crackles on auscultation. While listening to her chest you notice her heart sounds are quiet and discover her apex to be on the right-hand side.

What is the likely diagnosis and what else would you like to examine?

STATION 5

This station assesses your ability to elicit clinical signs:
- **Other**

This is a 9-minute station of clinical interaction. You will have up to 4 minutes beforehand to prepare yourself. No additional information will be given or is necessary before commencing the station. When the bell sounds you will be invited into the examination room.

INTRODUCTION

On entering the room you notice a young girl of 2 years. You are asked to inspect her arms and then go on to examine the relevant system.

CLINICAL SCENARIO

She appears well, although you suspect that she may have learning difficulties from her behaviour and apparent microcephaly. You notice in particular hypopigmented streaks and patches and cutaneous atrophy over her trunk and arms, and poor dentition.

Which system do you go on to examine?

What might you notice about her mother?

This station assesses your ability to assess specifically requested areas in a child with a developmental problem:
- Development

This is a 9-minute station of clinical interaction. You will have up to 4 minutes beforehand to prepare yourself. No additional information will be given or is necessary before commencing the station. When the bell sounds you will be invited into the examination room.

INTRODUCTION

You are asked to assess the vision of a 6-month-old infant. You are provided with a range of development assessment tools to aid you in your efforts.

CLINICAL SCENARIO

On initial inspection you do not notice any abnormality. The baby appears well grown and is sitting on his mother's lap with support. You take an object and offer it to the child but get no response. The child does not attempt to grab the object but when placed in his hands he does demonstrate a palmar grasp.

You then use a red ball to see if the child will fix and follow through 180° but get no response. The child fails to fix either on your face or that of the mother and there is only a brief interest on fixing to a light.

STATION 7

This station assesses your ability to communicate appropriate, factually correct information in an effective way within the emotional context of the clinical setting:

- **Communication One**

This is a 9-minute station consisting of spoken interaction. You will have up to 2 minutes before the start of the station to read this sheet and prepare yourself. You may make notes on the paper provided.

When the bell sounds you will be invited into the examination room. Please take this instruction sheet with you. The examiner will not ask questions during the 9 minutes but will warn you when you have approximately 2 minutes left.

You are not required to examine a patient.

The encounter should be focused on the task; you will be penalised for asking irrelevant questions or providing superfluous information. You will be marked on your ability to communicate, not the speed with which you convey information. You may not have time to complete the communication.

SETTING

You are a specialist registrar on a general ward of a district general hospital.

SCENARIO

You have been asked to speak to the parents of Oliver, a 2-year-old child with cerebral palsy. Oliver needs a cannula but is extremely difficult to gain access to. An SHO has had repeated attempts and despite parents' suggestions to ask for help the SHO continued regardless. Parents eventually became extremely angry and are demanding to speak to the consultant. They would like to take their child to another hospital.

BACKGROUND

Oliver was born at 25 weeks and had a very rocky time on the neonatal unit. He has suffered from sepsis, necrotising enterocolitis and required oxygen for his first year of life. He has severe developmental delay and is awaiting a gastrostomy/fundoplication to help him feed as he suffers from severe reflux. He has been admitted with gastroenteritis and is mildly–moderately dehydrated. He is not shocked but will require fluid therapy, which he has not tolerated by bolus nasogastric feed.

It is a weekend and the consultant is currently in consultation with the parents of a child with suspected non-accidental injury. He will not be available for at least 20 minutes.

This station assesses your ability to communicate appropriate, factually correct information in an effective way within the emotional context of the clinical setting:

- Communication Two

This is a 9-minute station consisting of spoken interaction. You will have up to 2 minutes before the start of the station to read this sheet and prepare yourself. You may make notes on the paper provided.

When the bell sounds you will be invited into the examination room. Please take this instruction sheet with you. The examiner will not ask questions during the 9 minutes but will warn you when you have approximately 2 minutes left.

You are not required to examine a patient.

The encounter should be focused on the task; you will be penalised for asking irrelevant questions or providing superfluous information. You will be marked on your ability to communicate, not the speed with which you convey information. You may not have time to complete the communication.

SETTING

You are a specialist registrar in a district general hospital.

SCENARIO

An 18-month-old child (Kate) has been admitted with a febrile convulsion. You must explain the diagnosis to the father. No further medical tests are necessary.

BACKGROUND

Kate had a viral upper respiratory tract infection and had a typical febrile convulsion (generalised, less than 5 minutes, complete neurological recovery). Examination of Kate was entirely normal and there are no features suggestive of meningitis or raised intracranial pressure. Kate does not require further tests and will be observed overnight for parental reassurance.

STATION 9

This station assesses your ability to take a focused history and explain to the parent your diagnosis or differential management plan:

- **History-taking and Management planning**

This is a 22-minute station of spoken interaction. You will have up to 4 minutes beforehand to prepare yourself. The scenario is below. Be aware that you should focus on the task given. You will be penalised for asking irrelevant questions or providing superfluous information. When the bell sounds you will be invited into the examination room. You will have 13 minutes with the patient (with a warning when you have 4 minutes left). You will then have a short period to reflect on the case while the patient leaves the room. You will then have 9 minutes with the examiner.

INFORMATION

You are a specialist registrar in a general paediatric clinic and receive the following letter from a GP regarding your next patient:

Dear Doctor

Re: Hisham Abbu

Age: 18 months

I would be grateful if you would see this young boy. His family have just moved into the area from Pakistan and from a brief letter I received from the family I believe he has a VSD. He is very small for his age and I am concerned about his growth. Thank you for your help in this matter.

Take a relevant history from Hisham's parents with regard to his potential problems. You do not need to examine Hisham or explain to the parents your management plan. You should be prepared to discuss this with the examiner.

DIAGNOSIS: PULMONARY STENOSIS (PS)

These findings suggest a diagnosis of pulmonary stenosis and in particular with the stenosis being at the level of the valve (in view of the click). In the exam diagnosis of this murmur would be entirely dependent on your being able to localise a systolic murmur to the pulmonary area. The click is an added bonus which will clinch the diagnosis but may not be picked up (apparently best heard at the third left intercostal space in expiration.) Textbooks also suggest the presence of a right ventricular heave (this will be felt at the *left* sternal border).

Pulmonary stenosis is an example of an acyanotic heart condition (critical pulmonary stenosis as a neonate has a different pathophysiology due to shunting and is a cyanotic heart condition). Do not forget to listen for a possible ventricular septal defect, which would indicate tetralogy of Fallot. Other valve or hole defects may also be present, e.g. atrial septal defect or patent ductus arteriosus in a more complicated cardiac lesion. Do not forget to look for a scar in the mid-axillary line; this may represent a scar after a Blalock–Taussig shunt (palliative procedure).

Important differentials to exclude are an atrial septal defect (also an ejection systolic murmur in the pulmonary area but you should hear a wide, fixed, split second heart sound – heard only by experts!) and aortic stenosis (louder in the aortic region and generally associated with a carotid or suprasternal thrill). There may be a suprasternal thrill with PS; a carotid thrill is diagnostic of aortic stenosis. If the murmur is soft, with no radiation, consider the possibility that this is an innocent pulmonary flow murmur.

Please see table below for investigations and management of PS.

NOONAN'S SYNDROME

This syndrome shares many phenotypic similarities with Turner's syndrome but can occur in both sexes. It can be inherited in an autosomal dominant pattern – chromosome 12q.

Classic features include:

- Short stature
- Facial dysmorphism, e.g. hypertelorism, down-slanting palpebral fissures, webbed neck, triangular facies, ptosis
- Cardiac defect (50%)
- Learning difficulties
- Chest deformities – pectus excavatum/carinatum.

Other features also include:

- Scoliosis
- Hepatosplenomegaly

Pulmonary stenosis

Investigations:	
CXR	Often normal but may see a prominent pulmonary artery or decreased pulmonary vascular markings in more severe disease
ECG	Normal if mild. If moderate to severe – right axis deviation and right ventricular hypertrophy In Noonan's you get a superior axis
ECHO	A gradient of >40 mmHg would indicate a need for surgery or the right ventricular pressure is >60 mmHg
Management:	
Multidisciplinary	Cardiologist, local paediatrician – local and tertiary referral centre
Conservative/medical	Adequate nutrition and growth May only need clinical review and no need for surgery if mild May need diuretics if associated significant shunts Need alprostadil (PGE1) in the presence of cyanotic congenital heart disease during the neonatal period Prophylaxis during surgical procedures
Surgical	Cardiac catheterisation Balloon valvuloplasty is the corrective treatment of choice
Associated conditions include:	Noonan's syndrome Tetralogy of Fallot

- Genitourinary anomalies
- Joint laxity
- Seizures
- Sensorineural hearing loss
- Bleeding disorders.

Investigations into the various associated conditions are required, e.g. cardiac work-up, renal ultrasound, audiometry and development. This should all be managed with a multidisciplinary team involving:

- Hospital professionals (paediatrician, cardiologist, ophthalmologist, neurologist, physiotherapist, occupational therapist, geneticist);
- Community professionals (paediatrician, GP, health visitor, community nurses).

Tetralogy of Fallot

Definition	1. VSD 2. Right ventricular hypertrophy 3. Right ventricular outlet obstruction 4. Overriding aorta This is an example of a cyanotic cardiac lesion. If the right ventricular outlet obstruction is mild these babies are often referred to as 'pink Fallots' as they have saturations in the normal range It represents approximately 8–10% of cardiac lesions in the UK
Symptoms	• 'Blue' baby • Failure to thrive • Dyspnoea on exertion • Cyanotic spells
Signs	• Cyanosis • Clubbing • Right ventricular heave • Systolic murmur/thrill, left lower sternal border • Single S2 • May have an aortic click
Risk factors/conditions	Fetal alcohol syndrome Maternal PKU Maternal antiepileptic use (e.g. carbamazepine) Di George's syndrome
CXR	'Boot-shaped' heart – uplifting of apex secondary to right ventricular hypertrophy Normal heart size Decreased pulmonary vascular markings
ECG	Right atrial hypertrophy Right ventricular hypertrophy Right axis deviation
Acute management	If presenting with a cyanotic spell: • Knee–chest position (baby) or encourage squatting • Morphine These actions reduce venous return and increase systemic vascular resistance. Right to left shunting (via increase in left-sided pressure) is reduced, improving pulmonary blood flow
Long-term management – medical	Multidisciplinary team Endocarditis prophylaxis Keep haematocrit <60%
Surgery	Palliative surgery, e.g. Blalock–Taussig shunt Total surgical correction

REMINDER

Areas to examine other than the heart in a cardiovascular assessment:

- *Colour*:
  - Pale (i.e., anaemic):
    - Conjunctiva
    - Palmar creases (compare your palm to the child's)
  - Blue:
    - Tongue (even if the lips show barn door cyanosis)
    - Fingertip and nail-bed (poor peripheral circulation not necessarily cyanosis)
- *Hands*: clubbing
- *Teeth*: evidence of caries?
- *Face*: dysmorphic features
- *Chest*:
  - Look, look, look for scars!
  - Effort of breathing
- *Pulses*: brachial and femoral bilaterally; look for femoral line scars
- *Blood pressure*.

COMMENTS ON STATION 2

DIAGNOSIS: HUNTER'S SYNDROME

'On examining Josh I note an appearance suggestive of a mucopolysaccharide storage disorder, as evidenced by his facies, short stature, bilateral hearing aids, thoracolumbar kyphosis and hepatosplenomegaly, and a scar suggestive of a left inguinal hernia operation. The most likely diagnosis is Hunter's syndrome as I saw no evidence of corneal clouding.'

The mucopolysaccharidoses (MPS) are a group of inherited disorders due to defects in glycosaminoglycan metabolism and are lysosomal disorders. Be familiar with the features of these disorders as these young people are often available for examinations.

The inability to degrade certain macromolecules results in their storage in a large variety of tissues, e.g. liver, spleen, heart and connective tissue. The precise clinical features of each MPS depend upon the specific enzymatic deficiency and the pattern of storage of the particular MPS. In addition to somatic features, which may be severe, significant learning difficulties occur in some groups of MPS. Diagnosis for all MPS may be made initially by measuring glycosaminoglycans in the urine and then enzymatic assay of white cells or cultured fibroblasts.

To date nine different types of MPS have been described. The main four are:

1. MPS I
   a. Hurler
   b. Schie

2. MPS II – Hunter
3. MPS III – Sanfilippo (severe neurological problems)
4. MPS IV – Morquio (usually normal intelligence).

The following summary of Hunter's and Hurler's is provided for the purist who is keen to know the difference and is confident of remembering the difference in the exam. It may be better for some candidates to be happy they know how to recognise children with MPS rather than get flustered on which one has corneal clouding.

- *Hu*nter's: **n**o corneal clouding (a **hunter** needs to **see** his **prey**)
- *Hurler's*: corneal clouding (a **hurler** doesn't!)

HUNTER'S SYNDROME

Hunter's syndrome is an X-linked recessive disorder caused by lack of the enzyme iduronate sulfatase. Onset of the disease is usually during the toddler years. Features include:

- Coarse facial features
- Skeletal irregularities: thoracolumbar kyphosis, scoliosis, short stature, joint stiffness, hernias, claw hand, thick skull
- Respiratory: obstructive airway
- Neurological: communicating hydrocephalus, macrocephaly, progressive hearing loss
- Ophthalmological: retinal degeneration (but no corneal clouding), retinitis pigmentosa
- Abdominal: hepatosplenomegaly
- Dermatological: white skin lesions may be found distributed symmetrically between the angles of the scapulae and posterior axillary lines, hypertrichosis, large tongue and thick lips
- Cardiac: valvular lesions
- Neurological: development regression, carpal tunnel syndrome.

There is no medical cure for the disease, although gene therapy may be a treatment of the future. Management involves a multidisciplinary team and treatment of symptoms, e.g. carpal tunnel surgery and genetic counselling.

HURLER'S SYNDROME

This is an autosomal recessive condition arising due to insufficient or absent levels of the enzyme α-L-iduronidase.

Features of this disorder are very similar to Hunter's syndrome – in facial features, organ enlargement and skeletal and developmental features. Differences include:

- Corneal clouding
- Language skills are poorer – secondary to hearing difficulties, large tongue and impaired vision

- Poor prognosis with cardiorespiratory problems making survival into the second decade unlikely.

Diagnosis (for Hunter's as well) is via increased levels of the glyco-saminoglycans heptan and dermatan sulfate in urine. There is also no cure for this disorder. Management within a multidisciplinary team is essential. There is a body of evidence that bone marrow transplants may change the disease process in Hurler's syndrome. Short cases and history-taking stations should focus on the multidisciplinary team approach unless you have detailed personal knowledge of novel treatments.

CAN YOU ...

Describe Tanner's scale for pubertal assessment?
   Obviously you are not out to embarrass any teenage participant in the exam but a good working knowledge may be useful, especially in the history and management planning station.

Female breast	Male genital	Pubic hair
1. Pre-pubertal	Pre-pubertal	Nil
2. Breast bud 8–13 years	Growth and texture change 10–13.5 years	Sparse and straight F: 8–14 years M: 10–15 years
3. Juvenile smooth contour	Length and girth growth	Coarser and curlier
4. Areola projects above breast	Darkening of scrotal skin	Adult type
5. Adult 12.5–18.5 years	Adult 14.5–18 years	Adult distribution F: 12.5–16.5 M: 14.5–18

Although not in the original definition, the appearance of axillary hair usually occurs in mid-puberty, approximately 2 years after the development of pubic hair.

COMMENTS ON STATION 3

DIAGNOSIS: LEFT HEMIPLEGIA WITH VENTRICULOPERITONEAL SHUNT

If while running through the station you forgot to check or ask to check the head circumference, you will struggle to pass – no matter how good your summary of events. Be warned!

'On examination I note evidence of a ventriculoperitoneal shunt and left hemiplegia as evidenced by paucity of movement on that side, with increased tone and brisk reflexes. Examples of causes would include previous periventricular, subarachnoid or subdural haemorrhage, congenital abnormality or previous meningitis. I would like to measure the child's head circumference and plot it on the child's growth chart.'

Observation is an essential part of the examination and will give a clue to the aetiological causes of the hemiparesis. Always inspect the back during the neurology examination as it is easy to miss spinal abnormalities that may accompany hydrocephalus, e.g. spina bifida. Other important comments:

- *Sutures*: open or closed?
- *Head shape*: is it symmetrical?
- *Hearing*: observed to startle to sounds?
- *Fundoscopy*: papilloedema? Difficult in the young infant but you must comment on the red reflex.

Important investigations would be cranial imaging (MRI and CT), but as the child already has a shunt it would be prudent to offer to take a thorough past medical history. This will force the examiner to either give you some vital clue (prematurity!) or change tack. For example, you may be asked in what situation you would rescan a child with a shunt. In this way you can score very good marks without ever coming to a definite diagnosis.

In performing a neurological examination in this age group it is essential to assess both central and peripheral tone. Initial impressions may be gathered by handling the baby and, if not already done, by undressing the child. To formally assess central tone, test for:

- *Head lag*: expect evidence of control from 6 weeks (pull the supine infant with both arms into the sitting position).
- *Sitting position*: assess ability to sit unsupported and stability in this position, which reflects truncal tone.
- *Standing position*: assess tone with support and, if able, without support.
- *Ventral suspension*: floppy or stiff? Are the arms and legs appropriately flexed?

With practice these movements can be performed one after the other by pulling up to sit, then stand and finally positioning ventrally. This looks very professional and is worth practising.

Peripheral tone is assessed in a similar manner to that in the older child. Assess whether floppy or reduced and to contrast look for evidence of spasticity and clonus. The scissoring of lower limbs when held upright is an indicator of increased tone.

Management involves a multidisciplinary approach:

Neurosurgical	Shunt management – revisions Risk of shunt infections
Neurological	Increased risk for seizures
Development	Paediatric assessment Physiotherapy Occupational therapy Social input and support groups GP
Coexisting pathology	E.g. cause of hydrocephalus might be post-ventricular haemorrhage secondary to extreme prematurity and so there may be other problems such as chronic lung disease

CAN YOU ...

Name the signs and symptoms of raised intracranial pressure (commonest reason for rescanning a shunt)? Remember you may have to do a shunt series to check for any breakages in the shunt. In children with long-term shunts the surrounding fibrosis may make the shunt break difficult to feel.

- At presentation:
  - Vomiting
  - Irritability
  - Poor feeding
  - Lethargic
  - (increased) seizures
  - Distended scalp veins
  - Sunsetting eyes.
- Without shunt revision (i.e., later signs):
  - Cushing's triad: bradycardia; hypertension; abnormal respiratory pattern
  - Decerebrate posture
  - Coma
  - Cardiorespiratory arrest.

COMMENTS ON STATION 4

DIAGNOSIS: KARTAGENER'S SYNDROME

An essential trait for a good paediatrician is empathy and being able to establish a good rapport with the patient. In this case it is important to understand and respect this young girl's modesty, but at the same time be able to ascertain the diagnosis. Being chatty during the examination may help gain her confidence, and will certainly calm your nerves. Although not formally examined this will be something the examiners will notice.

The examination findings are compatible with the diagnosis of bronchiectasis and the likely cause is Kartagener's syndrome with dextrocardia. It is important to include location of the apex beat as part of the respiratory examination, and missing dextrocardia would mean failing this station. Routinely examining for tracheal position and apex position will give you an overall idea about mediastinal location. Having demonstrated dextrocardia, one would like to look for evidence of situs inversus, e.g. by location of the liver. Although these stations seem to be the stuff of exam legend, they definitely do crop up!

BRONCHIECTASIS

Bronchiectasis is a permanent irreversible destruction of airways as a result of obstruction and/or inflammation of the airway.

Symptoms	Chronic/productive cough >3 months Haemoptysis
Signs	Clubbing Hyperexpanded chest Harrison sulci Crackles/wheeze (which do not improve after a good cough)
Investigation	CXR: not specific but may see ring, line and 'tramline' shadows CT: dilated bronchi seen Bronchoscopy Investigating aetiology, e.g. sweat test
Management (MDT) medical, nursing, psychological, social, school	Regular chest physiotherapy Antibiotics – acute exacerbations Those who have an element of reactive airway disease may respond to bronchodilators and steroids
Surgery	Pulmonary segmental resection Transplant

KARTAGENER'S SYNDROME

This syndrome is an autosomal recessive condition classically defined as a triad of:

1. bronchiectasis
2. chronic sinusitis
3. situs inversus.

It is an example of a primary ciliary dyskinesia. These patients present with chronic upper and lower respiratory tract symptoms which result from ineffective mucociliary clearance. In the case of males ciliary dysfunction results in immotile sperm. Nasal potential differences or the saccharin test (saccharin or another substance is placed in the nose, and the speed of transport into the nasopharynx is measured to calculate mucociliary clearance) may be useful in the diagnosis, as are nasal brushings and examination under the electron microscope.

Management of lower respiratory problems will be similar to that with bronchiectasis. Tympanostomy tubes reduce conductive hearing loss and recurrent infections and surgery can relieve sinus symptoms.

COMMENTS ON STATION 5

DIAGNOSIS: INCONTINENTIA PIGMENTI

These findings are consistent with incontinentia pigmenti: an X-linked dominant disorder involving the skin, dentition and central nervous system. There is a wide spectrum in this disorder, with some only having skin lesions and others with significant learning difficulties.

You would go on to assess the central nervous system and inspect the mother's skin. Details of the different skin manifestations during the age of the individual are shown below.

Stage of skin disease	Description
1st	The first stage is the erythematous and vesicular stage. It may be present at birth or appear soon after and may last from a few weeks to a few months
2nd	This is the verrucous stage. There can be thick crusts or scabs with healing and areas of increased pigmentation. The extremities are involved almost exclusively. This stage typically lasts months, but rarely as long as a year
3rd	The third state is the hyperpigmented stage, in which the skin is darkened in a swirled pattern. It usually appears between 6 and 12 months of life. The heavy pigmentation tends to fade with age in most affected individuals
4th	This stage is the atrophic stage. These scars are often present before the hyperpigmentation has faded and are seen in adolescents and adults as pale, hairless patches or streaks. These are most easily seen when they are on the calf or in the scalp. Once most patients reach adulthood (late teens and beyond), the skin changes may have faded and may not be visible to the casual observer

Neurological problems include cerebral atrophy and developmental delay. This may include slow motor development, muscle weakness in one or both sides of the body and seizures. Patients are also likely to have visual problems, including strabismus, cataracts and severe visual loss. Dental problems are also common, including missing or peg-shaped teeth. Dystrophic nails may also be present.

It is important to offer genetic counselling to these families and manage these patients within a multidisciplinary team.

COMMENTS ON STATION 6

DIAGNOSIS: BLIND

This child demonstrates no evidence of a response to basic visual cues and suffers from optic atrophy. You are not expected in this station to make the diagnosis but you should offer to examine the eyes in full as you demonstrated that the child is blind. The vital thing to remember is not to provide any auditory clues. Using a rattle as a visual clue and telling the examiner the child can see because she follows it with her eyes will make it impossible to pass. It is also vital you have checked the red reflex.

A neat little test if only one eye is potentially affected is to test the contralateral eye's response to light. If the contralateral pupil constricts the cortical function is intact and signals must be reaching the brain. If the contralateral pupil only constricts on direct application of light then there must be some disruption to nerve flow to the brain. Does the child have a glass eye?

On fundoscopy the appearance of pale optic discs would confirm the diagnosis of optic atrophy. Referral to an ophthalmologist is imperative and investigations include visual evoked responses and CT imaging.

For children with partial or complete blindness a number of management options are available. Teachers skilled in looking after children with visual problems are invaluable in aiding assessment and teaching parents to provide as much stimulation as possible for the child. Support groups and the Royal National Institute for the Blind can provide contacts and information for families. Financial support may be provided through application for disability living allowance.

This station focuses on development. Although it may be tempting to discuss conditions in which visual impairment/blindness may be present, it is important to focus attention on the development aspects. It is important to know approximate visual developmental milestones that you may be able to test in the station:

- One month:
  - Fixes on mum's face
  - Preferential looking test (will look towards cards with multiple stripes rather than one)
- One and a half months:
  - Will follow through 90° but not 180° (performed at 90 cm using a standard 4 cm ball)
- Three months:
  - Follows through 180°
- Ten months:
  - Effective use of pincer grip with raisin-sized object
  - Looks for fallen objects

- Twelve months:
  - Effective use of pincer grip with 'hundreds and thousands'.

More information on visual assessment is found on page 219.

COMMENTS ON STATION 7

This is a quasi-real scenario from the author's own experience. There are obviously a number of issues here which must be addressed:

1. Need to apologise to parents.
2. Need to explain that this is a situation which should not have occurred and that the situation will be discussed at a clinical governance meeting to ensure it does not happen again.
3. It is important that a solution is found for Oliver in the meantime, as Oliver's health is the most crucial at this point.
4. The consultant is unavailable but will be available to speak to parents at a later point (do not give a definite time).
5. Transfer to another hospital at this point is not in Oliver's best interests and it is imperative his condition is stabilised as a priority. Oliver is your most important priority in this matter and that by stabilising his condition and so calming his parents it may be that a transfer is no longer requested. You may therefore say:

'It is important that Oliver is stabilised before we would consider sending him to another hospital. That decision must be made by the consultant, Dr Smith, who unfortunately due to his acute clinical workload cannot be here at this time. It is my intention to provide Oliver with a means of receiving fluid and ensuring his adequate hydration. At that stage it will be possible to speak to Dr Smith about his subsequent care.'

Obviously the parents are going to be very upset and empathising with their frustration is paramount. They should not be allowed to be abusive (although this is unlikely to happen in the communication station). The communication station should be about just that. You should not have to make clinical decisions although you may gain Brownie marks for suggesting that a continuous infusion via a nasogastric tube be commenced to ensure Oliver's hydration. It may be that there was little clinical need for the cannula in the first place and you must indicate to the parents that you will examine Oliver to assess this. This must be done sensitively as, although the SHO has overstepped the mark, you do not want to imply that he is clinically incompetent.

The examiner will be looking to see you have:

- *sincerely* apologised;
- *allowed* parents to vent their frustration at the situation;
- *effectively* listened to their concerns about Oliver's present condition;
- *kindly but firmly* explained that the consultant is not available at this point but will speak to them when he is free;

- explained you *understand* that cannulation may prove to be very difficult so you will review Oliver's fluid requirements and provide a solution which causes Oliver the least distress;
- ensured that a management plan for further episodes will be placed in the notes to avoid similar incidents.

Appreciating the key communication points is only one step. The examiner must come away with the impression you are a compassionate doctor. Practice role-play with feedback is vital, as some candidates may not be as parent friendly as they think. A few tips are:

- Do not sit straight across from the parents – this creates an immediate barrier.
- Do not sit with your arms crossed.
- Lean forward, but not into their personal space.
- Give the parents time to express themselves. This may mean a few uncomfortable pauses.
- Ask the parents if you have addressed all their concerns.

This is a challenging station but if performed effectively the role-players are likely to have given you feedback just by their demeanour at the end of the scenario.

COMMENTS ON STATION 8

Most people will have experience of explaining what a febrile convulsion is and how to manage one (if you haven't, make sure you have!). In this scenario the key is to assume that a febrile convulsion is the worst experience a parent has had with their child. Be prepared to answer questions relating to the risks of epilepsy, as this is commonly asked.

General information on febrile convulsions:

- They are common (1 in 20).
- Often there is a family history.
- Typically 6 months to 3 years (although up to 6 years).
- Always in the presence of fever (and therefore infection).
- Risk of recurrence, especially the younger the child.
- Risk of epilepsy in later life is small (1%) and related to persistent febrile convulsions.

You might need to give parents a brief explanation of what they can do at home:

- If they recognise their child has a fever – to bring the temperature down, strip the child, provide a fan, give an antipyretic. You must emphasise that regular paracetamol will not stop their child having a febrile convulsion; also avoid being an advocate of 'fever phobia'.
- If the child has already started fitting – to ensure the environment is safe and to lay the child in the recovery position. Most seizures last less

than a couple of minutes but if it lasts longer than this to call for help (ambulance/GP).

- In the child with recurrent febrile convulsions where no other aetiology is found, a supply of buccal midazolam or rectal diazepam could be provided to give if the fits last longer than 5 minutes.

The role-player's statement (i.e., the father) contained the following information:

> *You are very worried as the last person you saw fit was your elderly father who later died of a brain tumour.*

Obviously this will add to the anxiety of the station. You must be prepared to answer questions relating to brain tumours and, presumably, 'Can my child have a scan?'. Scanning this child is entirely unjustified and you will be marked down for agreeing to tests which are not clinically needed. It is important to explain the differences between the child and the father's father. It is helpful to provide criteria for when we do scan (so that the father appreciates he is not just being fobbed off). For some families it is worth mentioning that every scan does contain radiation, which increases the risk of developing a tumour – although in this case that might be seen as rather callous!

COMMENTS ON STATION 9

The key areas to focus on in this scenario are the heart abnormality and concerns regarding growth and therefore the nutrition of the child. A suggested scheme:

1. Full history concerning the cardiac abnormality:
   a. Antenatal information
   b. When was the lesion diagnosed and what can they tell you about it?
   c. Cardiology input
   d. Medication
   e. Has there been a need for surgery and where was this done?
   f. Has the child ever been in heart failure?
2. Nutrition, growth and diet:
   a. Has the child had a trial of high-energy feeds?
   b. Diet history
   c. Has the child seen a dietician?
   d. Do they have any records of his previous heights and weights?
3. Drug history – particularly with reference to diuretics, ACE inhibitors.
4. Family history – is there consanguinity?
5. Other:
   a. Do the parents know about the importance of good dental hygiene?
   b. Are the parents aware that antibiotic prophylaxis is necessary?

What are the surgical options available? This may be asked by the parent.

As a first-year registrar you should be competent to explain the main surgical strategies and when they would be instituted.

Surgery is reserved for moderate to large VSDs, as small lesions are likely to close spontaneously. An echocardiogram will define the size of the lesion, although other signs at presentation – apical diastolic murmur, plethora and clubbing – are evidence of a large shunt. Failure of medical therapy when used for a moderate shunt will also prompt consideration of surgery. Ultimately surgery is used to prevent the complications of pulmonary hypertension. The pulmonary pressure (right-sided) is compared to aortic (systemic) and a ratio of greater than 2:1 is used as a rough guideline for the need for surgical intervention. The importance of an adequate weight prior to surgery should be emphasised.

Circuit F

STATION 1

This station assesses your ability to elicit clinical signs:

- CVS

This is a 9-minute station of clinical interaction. You will have up to 4 minutes beforehand to prepare yourself. No additional information will be given or is necessary before commencing the station. When the bell sounds you will be invited into the examination room.

INTRODUCTION

On entering the station you are presented with a 5-year-old child. You are told to examine his cardiovascular system.

CLINICAL SCENARIO

The young boy looks well. Peripheral examination is normal. Auscultation of the precordium reveals a soft systolic murmur at the upper left sternal edge. There are no scars, no thrills or heaves or radiation of the murmur. You note that the murmur disappears on changes of position.

How do you present your findings?

STATION 2

This station assesses your ability to elicit clinical signs:

- **Abdo/Other**

This is a 9-minute station of clinical interaction. You will have up to 4 minutes beforehand to prepare yourself. No additional information will be given or is necessary before commencing the station. When the bell sounds you will be invited into the examination room.

INTRODUCTION

On entering the room the examiner asks for your comments about a 4-month-old child.

CLINICAL SCENARIO

There is a well-nourished but small-for-age infant lying at rest on the bed. He is fully clothed but his head appears slightly jaundiced. You mention this to the examiner but bear in mind he has some dysmorphic features you cannot definitely identify.

The examiner asks you to look at his abdomen, but not palpate it. There is a scar in the right hypochondrium.

You tell the examiner you are suspicious of biliary atresia as there is evidence of an operation: presumably a Kasai procedure has been performed.

Instead of congratulating you on your clinical skills the examiner says, 'Bedside diagnosis already? Well then, can you listen to the child's precordium and tell me what you find?'.

You listen to the child's heart, wondering why, as this is an abdominal station, and are surprised to hear a murmur in the pulmonary area.

What murmur is this?

What condition does this child have?

STATION 3

This station assesses your ability to elicit clinical signs:
- **Neurological**

This is a 9-minute station of clinical interaction. You will have up to 4 minutes beforehand to prepare yourself. No additional information will be given or is necessary before commencing the station. When the bell sounds you will be invited into the examination room.

INTRODUCTION

You are asked to examine the peripheral nervous system of Jasmine, a 14-year-old girl.

CLINICAL SCENARIO

On inspection you notice that Jasmine has a tired expression, bilateral ptosis and is only in early puberty. Her proximal muscles, in particular, appear wasted but there is no fasciculation. Her tone appears normal, as do her reflexes. She is able to lift her arm up to shake your hand but her grip is weak. You proceed to test repetitive movement by asking her to imitate you making opening/closing movements of your hands. On repeated testing of her power you find she can lift her forearm from the bed but not against resistance.

What is the power grade (MRC) of her arm?

What is the most likely diagnosis?

STATION 4

This station assesses your ability to elicit clinical signs:
- **Respiratory/Other**

This is a 9-minute station of clinical interaction. You will have up to 4 minutes beforehand to prepare yourself. No additional information will be given or is necessary before commencing the station. When the bell sounds you will be invited into the examination room.

INTRODUCTION

On entering the room you are presented with a child approximately 6 months old. You are asked to examine Simon's respiratory system.

CLINICAL SCENARIO

You notice a plump but small-for-age child receiving oxygen via nasal cannulae. The child is plagiocephalic. His chest is hyperexpanded with normal vesicular breath sounds on examination. You note a small scar over the left lateral chest.

How will you present your findings and conclusion to the examiner?

STATION 5

This station assesses your ability to elicit clinical signs:

- **Other**

This is a 9-minute station of clinical interaction. You will have up to 4 minutes beforehand to prepare yourself. No additional information will be given or is necessary before commencing the station. When the bell sounds you will be invited into the examination room.

INTRODUCTION

You are asked to examine the eyes of a 13-year-old boy. His mother and sister are also in the room. His sister is in a wheelchair.

CLINICAL SCENARIO

On initial inspection you notice he is not dysmorphic, does not have ptosis or obvious ophthalmoplegia. You note he has brown eyes but no Kayser–Fleischer rings. He has normal acuity, pupils, visual fields, fundi and eye movements. You are then asked to compare his eyes to those of his sister and finally to look closely at his eyes in the light – you note blue sclerae.

What would you ask to examine next?

STATION 6

This station assesses your ability to assess specifically requested areas in a child with a developmental problem:

- **Development**

This is a 9-minute station of clinical interaction. You will have up to 4 minutes beforehand to prepare yourself. No additional information will be given or is necessary before commencing the station. When the bell sounds you will be invited into the examination room.

INTRODUCTION

On entering the room you see a bench containing a range of development assessment tools. You are asked to assess the speech and language of Matthew, a young boy of pre-school age.

CLINICAL SCENARIO

You introduce yourself to the mother and child. The child is sat at the foot of his mother and playing with a Thomas the Tank engine. He is about 3–4 years of age. He does not respond to your introduction. You attempt to engage him in conversation but get minimal response from the child and certainly no eye contact. He appears absorbed in his play. You ask the mother to engage with him. You notice he responds to his mother, although he continues to have his back turned. After repeated requests he eventually turns around.

What do you do?

STATION 7

This station assesses your ability to communicate appropriate, factually correct information in an effective way within the emotional context of the clinical setting:

- **Communication One**

This is a 9-minute station consisting of spoken interaction. You will have up to 2 minutes before the start of the station to read this sheet and prepare yourself. You may make notes on the paper provided.

When the bell sounds you will be invited into the examination room. Please take this instruction sheet with you. The examiner will not ask questions during the 9 minutes but will warn you when you have approximately 2 minutes left.

You are not required to examine a patient.

The encounter should be focused on the task; you will be penalised for asking irrelevant questions or providing superfluous information. You will be marked on your ability to communicate, not the speed with which you convey information. You may not have time to complete the communication.

SETTING

You are a specialist registrar in paediatrics at a district general hospital.

SCENARIO

It is the day after a bank holiday weekend and the ward pharmacist informs you that a drug error has been made. Steven, 13, who is meant to be receiving weekly methotrexate for arthritis, has instead received a daily dose over the bank holiday weekend. Steven's mother is waiting in the parents' room and is aware a drug error has been made. She is understandably upset over the potential consequences.

You must counsel Steven and his mother about the drug error and discuss what will be done about it.

This station assesses your ability to communicate appropriate, factually correct information in an effective way within the emotional context of the clinical setting:

- **Communication Two**

This is a 9-minute station consisting of spoken interaction. You will have up to 2 minutes before the start of the station to read this sheet and prepare yourself. You may make notes on the paper provided.

When the bell sounds you will be invited into the examination room. Please take this instruction sheet with you. The examiner will not ask questions during the 9 minutes but will warn you when you have approximately 2 minutes left.

You are not required to examine a patient.

The encounter should be focused on the task; you will be penalised for asking irrelevant questions or providing superfluous information. You will be marked on your ability to communicate, not the speed with which you convey information. You may not have time to complete the communication.

SETTING

You are an SpR on the neonatal unit.

SCENARIO

You have been asked to counsel and advise the mother of Peter, a 2-week-old infant. Peter's Guthrie test had indicated congenital hypothyroidism and subsequent blood tests have confirmed this. You must explain the diagnosis, and discuss the potential problems and treatment options. The diagnosis is not in doubt and no further blood tests are needed.

BACKGROUND

Peter's hypothyroidism was picked up by the normal screening process. Unfortunately, when he was brought to the unit for confirmation bloods there was a communication error between the SHO and the mother, who was told the results were normal (a patient with a similar surname had normal electrolyte results). When the consultant was told the result was normal he immediately asked for blood tests to be repeated as the child looked clinically hypothyroid. You have heard at a previous morning handover that the mother had been upset about the process.

STATION 9

This station assesses your ability to take a focused history and explain to the parent your diagnosis or differential management plan:

- **History-taking and Management planning**

This is a 22-minute station of spoken interaction. You will have up to 4 minutes beforehand to prepare yourself. The scenario is below. Be aware that you should focus on the task given. You will be penalised for asking irrelevant questions or providing superfluous information. When the bell sounds you will be invited into the examination room. You will have 13 minutes with the patient (with a warning when you have 4 minutes left). You will then have a short period to reflect on the case while the patient leaves the room. You will then have 9 minutes with the examiner.

INFORMATION

You are a specialist registrar in a district general hospital. You receive the following letter from a GP:

Dear Doctor

Re: Constance Patten

Age: 4

I would be grateful if you would see this young girl regarding constipation. I have previously prescribed laxatives but her mother has found that these have not helped. I would be grateful for your assistance, especially as Constance is now soiling and her mother is keen to solve this issue before she starts full-time primary school.

Take a thorough history from Constance's mother and explain your management plan to her.

COMMENTS ON STATION 1

DIAGNOSIS: INNOCENT MURMUR

> *'Jason is a well-grown boy and I would like to confirm this by plotting his height and weight on a growth chart. I note a soft, short systolic murmur grade 2/6 in the left upper sternal edge, which disappears on lying down, does not radiate and is not associated with a thrill or heave. Peripheral pulses are present. This is likely to be an innocent murmur.'*

On auscultating a murmur it is important to describe it adequately such that you describe all the features heard and lead neatly to the final diagnosis. This includes commenting on the location, radiation, grade and duration within the cardiac cycle. The classification of grades is found on page 111.

Innocent murmurs are common in general paediatric practice and therefore you should be prepared to have this diagnosis in your differential. Be aware of the different types of innocent murmurs, e.g. pulmonary flow murmur, venous hum and Still's murmur, and also the key features of 'normal murmurs'. If there is any suspicion then a murmur should always be investigated, by ECG, chest X-ray and – the gold standard – an echocardiogram.

FEATURES OF INNOCENT MURMURS – MODIFIED 'S' TEST

Soft **S**hort **S**ystolic **S**ymptom-free murmur over a **S**mall area which doesn't change on **S**itting or **S**tanding.

Signs (pulses) and **S**pecial investigations (ECG, CXR) are normal.

CAN YOU …

Explain to anxious parents what a diagnosis of an innocent murmur means?

Examples of innocent murmurs

Murmur	Features
Stills' murmur	Early soft systolic Lower left sternal edge
Pulmonary flow murmur	Soft ejection systolic 2nd left intercostal space
Venous hum	Continuous systolic Right clavicle

COMMENTS ON STATION 2

DIAGNOSIS: ALAGILLE'S SYNDROME

If you have an Aspergeresque memory then Alagille's is an autosomal dominant disorder owing to mutations in the JAG1 gene on chromosome 20p12. JAG1 codes for a NOTCH receptor ligand important in cell–cell interactions and in development. Different mutations have been described, 70% of which are sporadic.

It is much more important to remember some of the key features. Alagille's syndrome is characterised by a paucity of interlobular bile ducts (intrahepatic cholestasis).

The classic syndrome consists of:

1. Jaundice in early infancy (and chronic cholestasis)
2. Characteristic facies (prominent forehead, chin and nasal bridge, deep-set eyes, upward sloping palpebral fissures)
3. Pulmonary stenosis
4. Butterfly vertebrae
5. Growth and mental retardation
6. Ocular anomalies, e.g. posterior embryotoxon-opaque border to cornea.

In this case the scar was for a liver biopsy, not a Kasai procedure. The murmur was an ejection systolic murmur typical of pulmonary stenosis. Examination would have been completed by examining the back for evidence of vertebral abnormalities and looking for evidence of scratch marks on the skin (the pruritus is intense).

Treatment is with cholestyramine (for the itch) and phenobarbital. Liver transplants may be needed for severe cholestasis.

REMINDER

A HIDA scan is used to differentiate between intra- and extrahepatic causes of cholestasis. Infants need phenobarbital prescribed for approximately 5 days before this investigation (easy to remember; looks good if you get asked).

CAN YOU …

Describe the appearance of these scars?

- Kasai
- Liver biopsy
- Liver transplant (classically a 'Mercedes Benz scar')
- Cholestectomy (laparoscopic/open)
- Pyloroplasty.

See Figure 4 on page 89.

DIAGNOSIS: MYASTHENIA GRAVIS

The presence of bilateral ptosis makes a myopathy a more likely diagnosis. Myopathies are neuromuscular disorders in which the primary symptom is muscle weakness. Myopathies can be inherited or acquired. They may be categorised into:

- Congenital myopathies
- Muscular dystrophies
- Mitochondrial myopathies
- Glycogen storage diseases of muscle
- Dermatomyositis
- Myositis ossificans
- Polymyositis.

Exclude a dystonia (e.g. myotonic dystrophy) by shaking hands with the patient. A dystonia is a neurological movement disorder characterised by sustained muscle contractions, usually producing twisting and repetitive movements or abnormal postures or positions.

In the presence of reduced power exclude myasthenia gravis by demonstrating fatiguability (loss of strength upon exertion that improves after rest). A suitable answer would be:

'On examining Jasmine she appears young for her age and I would like to confirm this by plotting her height and weight on the appropriate growth chart. Neurologically I noted an expressionless facies, bilateral ptosis and demonstrated fatiguability on assessing her power. There was no evidence of dystonia and reflexes were normal. I would like to complete my examination by examining her eye movements and assessing her cranial nerves. The most likely diagnosis is myasthenia gravis.'

This is a rare disorder but by thinking systematically and by demonstrating assessment of fatiguability you are showing your thinking. Mentioning growth and delayed puberty shows knowledge regarding chronic disorders.

Myasthenia gravis is a disorder resulting in progressive muscle weakness. It arises due to reduced acetylcholine transfer/receptiveness across the neuromuscular junction. In the neonatal period this may arise due to inherited defect of the acetylcholine receptor or to transplacental transfer of the immunoglobulin from the mother suffering from myasthenia gravis.

Juvenile myasthenia is an autoimmune disease. In this age group, symptoms commonly involve the ocular muscles but can affect the lower cranial nerves and respiratory muscles.

Treatment should be part of a multidisciplinary team involving liaison between neurologist, local paediatrician, school and GP.

Investigations	
Anti-AChR antibodies assay	Positive in approximately 50% of patients
Anticholinesterase test (Tensilon test)	Administration of edrophonium
EMG	Repetitive nerve stimulation (RNS) should lead to a decremental response in compound action potentials on EMG
Muscle biopsy	Fewer acetylcholine receptors on histological analysis
CT/MRI	Look for evidence of thymoma
Other	Autoantibodies Consider thyroid function looking for evidence of other autoimmune disease

Treatment	
Anticholinesterase medication	Pyridostigmine
Immunosuppressants	Steroids, azathioprine, ciclosporin
Plasmapheresis	
Intravenous immunoglobulin	
Thymectomy	

CAN YOU …

Correctly use the MRC power scale?

Like the classification of murmurs, the assessment of power is very precise. It is important that what you say and what you find are one and the same. If a child can raise their arm off the bed, no matter how weak they are, they must have power of at least 3.

- 0 No contraction
- 1 Flicker of contraction
- 2 Active movement in a plane perpendicular to gravity
- 3 Active movement against gravity
- 4 Movement against resistance
- 5 Normal power

Do not use terms like 4+, unless you were a paediatric neurologist in a former life.

DIAGNOSIS: CHRONIC LUNG DISEASE

> *'On examining Simon I notice he has supplemental oxygen of 1l/min via nasal cannulae. He appears small and I would like to confirm this by plotting his length, weight and head circumference on a growth chart, correcting for gestational age. On assessment of his respiratory system I note he is hyperexpanded as evidenced by an increased anterior–posterior diameter. There is no evidence of crackles or wheeze. I also noted a lateral thoracotomy scar, which suggests ligation of a persistent ductus arteriosus. These findings suggest a diagnosis of chronic lung disease.'*

In this age group the diagnosis of chronic lung disease is the most likely. Patients will not always have clinical findings on auscultation but nevertheless you should use this time to formulate your answer to the examiner. Chronic lung disease is currently defined as an oxygen dependency at 36 weeks post-conceptional age. Look for other clues associated with prematurity.

	Tips
Exam	Look for other clues like scars • Chest drains • PDA ligation • VP shunt • Inguinal hernia repair • NEC scars/drains • Central lines May/may not be wheeze and crackles Growth and weight may be low
Management – Respiratory	Oxygen Prevention of infection – immunisation Medication • Inhaled steroids • Bronchodilators • Diuretics • Na/K/PO_4 supplements • Vitamins • Fe
Dietician	Optimise nutrition and supplements
Multidisciplinary team	Community and hospital (neonatologists/tertiary specialists/GP/health visitor/community paediatrician)

PERSISTENT DUCTUS ARTERIOSUS

This is a persistence of the fetal circulation connecting the pulmonary artery to the descending aorta and is more common in the premature infant. The table below summarises the key features.

History	If small there may be no symptoms Larger ducts result in symptoms of heart failure: • Breathlessness (especially during feeds) • Weight gain • Cough • Chest infections
Risk factors	Premature Low birth weight Maternal rubella Trisomies
Examination	Noted incidentally during admission on neonatal unit Continuous machinery murmur (or ejection systolic) radiating to the scapula/back Bounding pulses Wide pulse pressure Systolic thrill Signs of heart failure: • Gallop rhythm • Poor peripheral perfusion • Hepatomegaly • Tachypnoea • Tachycardia
Investigation	ECG CXR ECHO
Treatment – acute	Respiratory support Oxygen Diurectics Sodium and fluid restriction
Surgical	Coil embolisation Duct ligation (lateral thoracotomy scar)/thoracoscopic ligation
Medical	Prophylaxis for endocarditis In the pre-term infant consideration for the use of indometacin/ibuprofen

DIAGNOSIS: OSTEOGENESIS IMPERFECTA

The request to examine the eyes at this station was a clue regarding a diagnosis of osteogenesis imperfecta. Although time constraints prevented one author from demonstrating all these features, the examiner did agree the blue sclera were a soft sign and must have felt the candidate had demonstrated a competent eye examination as the candidate was awarded a good mark.

Do not be put off if you cannot identify positive signs. Examiners are aware that some patients will have soft signs and will guide you if signs are present. However, on occasion patients are provided who have no positive physical signs – do not be tempted to make something up!

Tips for examining eyes

Inspection	Squint Nystagmus Ptosis Swelling/red eye Glasses Kayser–Fleischer rings (Wilson's disease) Blue sclera (connective tissue disease) Other general features, e.g. growth, dysmorphism
Acuity	Snellen chart Reading
Pupils (test second and third cranial nerves)	Pupil size Light reflexes Accommodation reflexes Relative afferent papillary defect
Visual fields (second cranial nerve)	Use red marker/fingers
Eye movements (third, fourth and sixth cranial nerves)	Nystagmus Diplopia (and which image is lost on closing different eyes)
Cover test	Testing strabismus
Fundoscopy	Optic discs: • Optic atrophy • Papilloedema • Papillitis • Retinitis pigmentosa • Hypertension • Diabetic changes • Miscellaneous, e.g. cherry-red spot

OSTEOGENESIS IMPERFECTA

This musculoskeletal disorder results from an abnormality within collagen. Many forms have been described and may be inherited as autosomal dominant or recessive. The table below lists features common to the various types.

History	Easy bruising Fracture after trivial trauma Deafness Significant family history Antenatal fractures/limb shortening/miscarriages
Examination	Blue sclerae (not present in all types) Kyphoscoliosis Hearing aids Plaster casts/scars from fractures Joint hypermobility Short stature Dysmorphic facies (e.g. frontal bossing/triangular facies) Dentition anomalies
Investigation	Bone mineral density Other, e.g. skin biopsy culturing dermal fibroblasts Skeletal survey – fractures/healing fractures/osteopenia/broad bones
Treatment	Surgery • Scoliosis correction, e.g. intramedullary rodding Genetic counselling Parental education, e.g. optimal holding position of child; shock-absorbing footwear; orthotics No definitive medical treatment available

COMMENTS ON STATION 6

DIAGNOSIS: UNDERGOING INVESTIGATION FOR AUTISTIC SPECTRUM DISORDER

This is the nightmare situation for many candidates. You have been given a difficult task to begin with, which is made worse by the potential uncooperative nature of the child. Do not panic; take a deep breath and reiterate the instruction in your mind. The examiner will almost certainly share your anguish. The instruction was to assess the speech and language of a pre-school-age child. An approach to the station may be:

> 'At present Matthew appears not to want to be disturbed. The ability to hear is an important determinant of speech and language development. I do not see an obvious hearing aid and although slow to respond he did eventually acknowledge his mother. He appears older than 2 years of age so I would expect him to be able to use two- to three-word sentences. He may know his name and potentially some colours. May I ask his mother if he is able to do this?'

The examiners will either allow you to do this or they won't. If they do you will gain valuable information and it gives you a point to move on from. If the examiner is not keen for you to gain this information then you will need to interact with Matthew. It may be you find another train to bring alongside Matthew's, find some pens and crayons and start drawing in bold colours or maybe play a musical instrument. At some point Matthew, even if he doesn't speak, should show interest in your activities. To spend the entire station transfixed by one item would be abnormal behaviour for a school-age child. In fact if you removed the train from Matthew (with mother's permission) he would become extremely distressed.

This child *may* have autism. In a 5-minute session it is impossible to make a diagnosis of autism as this diagnosis requires good history-taking to assess for abnormalities in the areas of behaviour, language and social communication. In the development station certain key things may give one clues:

- Unusual ways of playing with toys and other objects, such as only lining them up a certain way.
- Lack of imagination in play.
- Repetitive body movements or patterns of behaviour, such as hand-flapping, spinning and head-banging.
- Hyperactive behaviour.
- Unusual use of pronouns, echolalia.

In the differential diagnosis of autism one should make attempts to ascertain whether the child can hear, e.g. making an obvious noise and assessing the response and observing how the child plays alone, with their mother and with the candidate.

Do not worry if you cannot fully engage with the child, as long as you demonstrate what you are trying to do. In an examination setting these are often difficult to elicit as the child will not be relaxed. The examiners are aware of this.

COMMENTS ON STATION 7

The following is an example of how to approach the situation:

1. Introduce yourself and explain that you have asked the named nurse also to attend and have made efforts not to be disturbed, e.g. cannot be bleeped.
2. Understanding of parents' awareness of situation.
3. Explain and apologise for the error.
4. Risk management to deal with error, i.e. notification of the critical incident (and that you will complete the form) and if they wish to take the matter further to involve the patient advisory liaison service.
5. Management regarding effects of medication: blood tests, side effects.
6. Answer any questions and, if they have further questions, you will address them.

These scenarios may have the added difficulty of the parent being irate – a reflection of what actually happens in clinical practice. Do not be put off by this approach. As long as you are calm, polite and actively listen you will be rewarded a good mark.

Methotrexate's potentially toxic effects are related to its interaction with the folic acid pathway. Side effects may be dose dependent or independent:

- Mouth sores – dose dependent
- Stomach upset (nausea, vomiting, diarrhoea) – dose dependent
- Liver toxicity – dose independent
- Pneumonitis – dose independent
- Bone marrow toxicity
- Headache
- Drowsiness
- Itchiness
- Skin rash
- Dizziness
- Hair loss
- Low white cell count.

Important blood tests include full blood count, liver function tests, urea and electrolytes and monitoring.

COMMENTS ON STATION 8

This is a potentially challenging station as, although the subject matter is not difficult to explain, the issue will be clouded by the mistake made. By now you should see that there is a very familiar pattern in the approach to answering the communication station. Once again:

- Introduce yourself with name *and* grade.
- Ensure you tell the mother you will not be disturbed.
- Ensure you ask if there is anyone else she would like to be present.
- Apologise for the error; be humble and explain the issue will be brought up in the next departmental meeting to stop things like this happening again.
- Ask the mother if she understands why she was brought back for bloods.
- Ask the mother if she has any understanding of the term *hypothyroidism* (any elderly relative might well be on thyroxine).
- Explain in general terms what the thyroid gland does.
- Explain the need for *lifelong* thyroxine and the reasons for this.
- Ask if she has any questions.

The above, even without any interruptions, should take you through to time easily. Remember that you do not have to complete all the tasks to pass the station. You will be assessed on what you say and how you say it. As long as you are not rambling you will only be penalised for irrelevancies. Do not get stuck on issues such as repeating bloods or the potential of thyroid transplant.

Do listen to the mother. She may be very angry with the initial misdiagnosis or she may be angry because she is scared (e.g. she may have related her mother's early death to her hypothyroidism; will her child die early?).

Show off some of your knowledge while talking:

'Although your child may look perfectly well without treatment, we can predict that in weeks or months his skin may become dry, feeding more difficult and his muscles more floppy. We know that without regular thyroxine his growth will be poor and his intellectual development slower than normal.'

The key features of congenital hypothyroidism are worth knowing:

- Growth failure and intellectual impairment
- Poor tone
- Decreased physical activity for the child's age
- Thick tongue
- Anaemia
- Umbilical hernia
- Constipation
- Hoarse cry
- Jaundice
- Coarse facies.

Treatment is with levothyroxine. Initially the child may be very responsive to thyroxine, so advise the mother that it may take some time to settle on a regular dose. It is important to emphasise the need to take regular thyroxine. You can imagine it is difficult to understand why you have to keep giving regular medication to a completely well child! Emphasising the risks of intellectual impairment (avoid the term retardation) is useful in this regard.

COMMENTS ON STATION 9

This is a very common problem – one you may already be familiar with. In this station you are expected to take a directed history and then discuss the management with the examiner.

The following is an example of an answer:

- Presenting complaint: how often bowels are opened; frequency of soiling; stool description; pain on defecation; abdominal pain/distension.
- Rule out organic causes: hypothyroidism or surgical, e.g. Hirschsprung's disease.
- Risk factors: diet (fibre and fluid intake).
- Birth history: meconium passed in first 24 hours; feeding and weaning.
- Past medical history/family history – clues to organic causes.
- Drug history – previous treatments of other medication impacting on constipation.
- Social history: family/nursery response to behaviour; strategies in toileting.

In feeding back to the examiner you may be asked to describe what you would write in your letter to the GP. It is essential not only to accumulate the information obtained in the history session but also to formulate the management plan. An important part of managing constipation is to explain to families that it is common; encourage behavioural, diet and medication strategies, and explain that there is no overnight solution.

Beware that in the history-taking you may uncover information that you may not relate directly to the presenting complaint. For example, one author found that in a history station a patient's father had recently been diagnosed with terminal colon cancer.

MANAGEMENT STRATEGIES

The three main strategies are:

- Empty the colon of stool.
- Establish regular soft and painless bowel movements.
- Maintain very regular bowel habits.

Conservative/behavioural methods	High-fibre diet Increase fluid intake Healthy diet (low sugar) Star charts/reward system Making the toilet a 'friendly place' Encourage regular routine involving sitting on the toilet for a period of time
Osmotic laxatives (soften stool)	Lactulose Polyethylene glycol
Stimulant laxatives (encourage motility)	Senna Picosulfate Docusate sodium
Enema	Empty bowel – by pushing fluid into rectum, softening stool and creating pressure in rectum to release stool
Suppositories	Glycerine – stimulating rectum to release stool

Side effects of laxatives include:

- Abdominal cramps
- Flatulence
- Belching
- Bloating
- Nausea
- Mild diarrhoea
- Thirst.

An approach used by this author includes commencing an osmotic laxative to soften the stool and then introducing a stimulant laxative to continue regular toileting. This should be done in conjunction with a behaviour strategy, e.g. star charts. In the case of the chronically constipated child a 'clear-out' would be more appropriate, e.g. a short course of polyethylene glycol laxative ('Movicol') or in more severe cases admission to hospital for an enema.

Movicol is becoming increasingly utilised as an agent in the fight against children who won't poo. As a sachet in a large volume of fluid, Movicol can be drunk over a period of time rather than in one go (as for a bowel prep). It would be worthwhile making sure you know your own local policy so that you can back up your particular management plan.

Circuit G

STATION 1

This station assesses your ability to elicit clinical signs:
- **CVS**

This is a 9-minute station of clinical interaction. You will have up to 4 minutes beforehand to prepare yourself. No additional information will be given or is necessary before commencing the station. When the bell sounds you will be invited into the examination room.

INTRODUCTION

On entering the room you are presented with a small infant. The examiner says, 'Please examine the cardiovascular system of this 3-week-old baby girl and present your findings'.

CLINICAL SCENARIO

On general inspection you note that the baby is not dysmorphic and is pink and well perfused. There is an obvious left-sided scar. The child is not attached to any monitoring and has no clinical signs of respiratory distress, clubbing or cyanosis. Interestingly, the left hand appears cooler than the right and when you come to examine the brachial pulses the left appears weaker. The heart rate is 140 beats per minute. There is no hepatomegaly and the femoral pulses are palpable with no radiofemoral delay.

The left-sided scar runs from just below the nipple backwards and inferiorly to beneath and behind the armpit. There is also a 1 cm scar just inferior to its lower border. On auscultation a long systolic murmur, without a thrill, is heard throughout the precordium, radiating to the back. The first and second heart sounds are normal, as are the breath sounds.

What defect does the cardiovascular findings suggest and what bedside test would be important to request?

As you present your findings you notice she has fat and puffy feet. Is this of significance and what other findings may be present on the examination?

This station assesses your ability to elicit clinical signs:
* Abdo/Other

INTRODUCTION

On entering the room you are asked to examine the abdominal system of a 10-year-old boy.

CLINICAL SCENARIO

On initial inspection you note a pale boy who has a rounded face and patchy loss of hair to his scalp. His conjunctivae are pale but there is no evidence of scleral jaundice. His mouth is normal with no ulcers. On asking him to remove his T-shirt you notice that he has a pouch hanging around his neck into which is placed the end of a dual-lumen catheter (one red, one white) tunnelled to the right upper chest. There are a few petechiae across his chest. Respiratory and pulse rate are within the normal range for age.

What differentials will you have in mind at this point? What else will you specifically examine in addition to the abdomen?

His abdomen is mildly distended without scars or venous abnormality but he does have obvious striae. His liver edge is palpable three finger-breadths below the costal margin and the spleen palpable four finger-breadths below the costal margin. The rest of the examination is normal.

How will you present these findings to the examiner?

What bedside information would you request from the examiner?

This station assesses your ability to elicit clinical signs:
- **Neurological**

This is a 9-minute station of clinical interaction. You will have up to 4 minutes beforehand to prepare yourself. No additional information will be given or is necessary before commencing the station. When the bell sounds you will be invited into the examination room.

INTRODUCTION

A well Afro-Caribbean girl is seated cooperatively on a chair. You are told, 'Please examine the eyes of this 6-year-old girl, who presented with morning vomiting'.

CLINICAL SCENARIO

On general inspection she is not dysmorphic. You examine in the following order:

- *Acuity*: Testing each eye individually (Snellen chart) – no defect.
- *Visual fields*: Testing each eye individually – no defect.
- *Eye movements*: You note that there is reduced lateral movement of the left eye. All other movements of both eyes are normal. The girl complains of diplopia on left lateral gaze. There is no nystagmus.
- *Squint*: You find that there is no tropia or phoria present.
- *Pupils*: The pupils are equal and reactive to light and accommodation.
- *Fundoscopy*: You find bilateral mild papilloedema (blurred disc margins and venous congestion) with no haemorrhage or exudates.
- *Eyelids*: No ptosis present.

What nerve(s) are involved to give this pattern of external ophthalmoplegia?

What is the most likely cause of the vomiting?

What are the causes of the above condition in children?

What would be your first-line investigations?

This station assesses your ability to elicit clinical signs:

- **Respiratory/Other**

INTRODUCTION

The examiner tells you that this 7-year-old child has presented to his GP many times with a nocturnal cough. Could you examine his respiratory system to find out why?

CLINICAL SCENARIO

The child appears well grown and is breathing comfortably at rest. You ask him to remove his T-shirt and sit up on the couch. On general inspection you note that he has mild respiratory distress (intercostal recession) with a respiratory rate of 35 per minute. He appears to have prominent chest musculature and Harrison's sulci bilaterally. He has no peripheral stigmata of respiratory disease, has a pulse rate of 90 beats per minute and is not centrally or peripherally cyanosed.

There is no palpable lymphadenopathy in the cervical or axillary regions. The chest has no scars. There is an apparent increased anteroposterior diameter when assessed from the side. You examine the front completely, followed by the back. There is bilateral equal expansion and resonant percussion note. There is a mild diffuse expiratory wheeze throughout the chest. There is no palpable liver edge.

What is the most likely diagnosis?

What part of the respiratory system examination should you offer to examine next?

What additional bedside tests are important in this child?

STATION 5

This station assesses your ability to elicit clinical signs:
- **Other**

This is a 9-minute station of clinical interaction. You will have up to 4 minutes beforehand to prepare yourself. No additional information will be given or is necessary before commencing the station. When the bell sounds you will be invited into the examination room.

INTRODUCTION

On entering the room you are invited to comment on the appearance of Crystal, a 6-year-old girl.

CLINICAL SCENARIO

Crystal is lying on the couch accompanied by her mother (who is wearing glasses and has multiple 'skin tags' apparent on her face). On general inspection Crystal has no striking abnormalities. You ask her to remove her vest and sit up for you. At this point you notice a number of brown pigmented patches with smooth outlines of variable size over her abdomen and chest.

You begin formal examination at the hands, moving up the arms to the axillae, which appear freckled. The face is not affected and there are no mucosal lesions in the mouth. The anterior and posterior aspects of the chest have multiple (> 5) pigmented patches present, with the largest measuring 10 × 15 cm approximately.

What is your current working diagnosis?

You present your findings so far to the examiner and explain that you wish to examine the child for associated features.

What systems will you now examine and how will you structure your examination?

STATION 6

This station assesses your ability to assess specifically requested areas in a child with a developmental problem:

- **Development**

This is a 9-minute station of clinical interaction. You will have up to 4 minutes beforehand to prepare yourself. No additional information will be given or is necessary before commencing the station. When the bell sounds you will be invited into the examination room.

INTRODUCTION

On entering the room, the examiner asks you to assess the motor development of an infant the Child Development Centre have been following up.

CLINICAL SCENARIO

The infant is accompanied by her mother. On initial general inspection you find her to be looking around lying on her back. She is moving all four limbs, is able to reach out for bright toys, pass objects from hand to hand and to place them in her mouth. She turns to her mother's voice but makes little noise and no words herself.

You ask the mother if you may examine her more closely. With permission you then formally test the motor development (gross and fine motor).

On pulling to sit there is reduced truncal tone and mildly reduced head control. She is unable to sit unsupported. When held vertically, she will put weight on both legs and bounce weakly. She will not support herself or hold on to the cot side for support. In ventral suspension you again note impaired head control (to 45°) and truncal hypotonia. On lying her down on her front the infant will push on her hands a limited amount. You move on to test the Moro reflex, which has been lost.

You test fine motor control initially with a single bright red brick, which she takes in a full palmar grasp and transfers from hand to hand. A second brick is introduced, which she takes in her other hand and then bangs the bricks together. She is not able to scribble with a crayon, build blocks into a tower of three or put pieces into a simple jigsaw.

What is the developmental age of this child in the area of gross motor development?

What is the developmental age of this child in the area of fine motor development?

What additional developmental reflexes could you describe or test in this child?

STATION 7

This station assesses your ability to communicate appropriate, factually correct information in an effective way within the emotional context of the clinical setting:

- Communication One

This is a 9-minute station consisting of spoken interaction. You will have up to 2 minutes before the start of the station to read this sheet and prepare yourself. You may make notes on the paper provided.

When the bell sounds you will be invited into the examination room. Please take this instruction sheet with you. The examiner will not ask questions during the 9 minutes but will warn you when you have approximately 2 minutes left.

You are not required to examine a patient.

The encounter should be focused on the task; you will be penalised for asking irrelevant questions or providing superfluous information. You will be marked on your ability to communicate, not the speed with which you convey information. You may not have time to complete the communication.

SETTING

You are the SpR at a district general hospital working in the outpatient clinic.

SCENARIO

Dean (12 years old) has been brought for review in clinic following a recent admission. Your task is to discuss with Dean and his mother the need for a regular inhaled steroid for control of his asthma. You should also confirm the family's understanding of the management plan for an acute exacerbation.

BACKGROUND

Dean was recently admitted for 5 days to the children's ward with a severe acute exacerbation of his asthma. Over the preceding 12 hours he had been using his salbutamol inhaler every 20 minutes at home with no improvement. In the emergency department he had required oxygen, salbutamol and ipratropium nebulisers, i.v. salbutamol and i.v. hydrocortisone in order to see improvement.

He had been discharged home with a short course of oral prednisolone and, as required, inhaled salbutamol by spacer. His mother had refused to start him on inhaled steroid at discharge but was happy to come to an outpatient appointment to discuss the options.

Dean was a normal term delivery and has a normal developmental history. He has no other medical problems and takes no other medication. He lives with his mother (a heavy smoker) and sister, both of whom suffer with eczema. He has a significant persistent night-time cough and daytime wheeze with exercise.

Do *not* take any further history.

You will not be asked any questions by the examiner, but you must be prepared to answer any questions from the patient or his mother. You may not discuss all the possible information in the time appointed but will be expected to cover individual areas in sufficient detail.

STATION 8

This station assesses your ability to communicate appropriate, factually correct information in an effective way within the emotional context of the clinical setting:

- **Communication Two**

This is a 9-minute station consisting of spoken interaction. You will have up to 2 minutes before the start of the station to read this sheet and prepare yourself. You may make notes on the paper provided.

When the bell sounds you will be invited into the examination room. Please take this instruction sheet with you. The examiner will not ask questions during the 9 minutes but will warn you when you have approximately 2 minutes left.

You are not required to examine a patient.

The encounter should be focused on the task; you will be penalised for asking irrelevant questions or providing superfluous information. You will be marked on your ability to communicate, not the speed with which you convey information. You may not have time to complete the communication.

SETTING

You are the SpR in a district general hospital working in a special care baby unit.

SCENARIO

You are presented with Donna, a 21-year-old in her first pregnancy, now at 24 weeks' gestation. She was admitted through the emergency department with lower abdominal cramps and vaginal fluid loss. She has been assessed by the obstetrician and given steroid as he feels she is at risk of pre-term delivery.

You have been asked to discuss with Donna and her partner Jamie the resuscitation and stabilisation of the baby if it is born at 24 weeks.

BACKGROUND INFORMATION

Donna was previously fit and well with no past medical problems. She is taking no regular medication and has no allergies. She had normal booking bloods including the triple test and normal booking and anomaly ultrasound scans.

You should not take any further medical history.

This station assesses your ability to take a focused history and explain to the parent your diagnosis or differential management plan:

- History-taking and Management planning

This is a 22-minute station of spoken interaction. You will have up to 4 minutes beforehand to prepare yourself. The scenario is below. Be aware that you should focus on the task given. You will be penalised for asking irrelevant questions or providing superfluous information. When the bell sounds you will be invited into the examination room. You will have 13 minutes with the patient (with a warning when you have 4 minutes left). You will then have a short period to reflect on the case while the patient leaves the room. You will then have 9 minutes with the examiner.

INFORMATION

You are the SpR in a paediatric outpatient clinic at a district general hospital. You have received the following referral letter from a GP:

Dear Doctor

Re: James X

I would be grateful if you could see this 5-year-old boy in your outpatient clinic with regard to his episodes of loss of consciousness. He has developed these episodes over the preceding 4 months and has been seen in the local emergency department on one occasion following an occurrence at school. A 12-lead ECG, BP, FBC, glucose and U&Es at this time were normal.

He was born by NVD at term and has shown normal development to date. He has no other past medical history and takes no medication. He has one elder sister (8 years), who was diagnosed with febrile convulsions at age 3 years and has had no further problems.

He has recently moved to a new school and his parents feel he has settled in well.

I wonder if he may have a seizure disorder or cardiac dysrhythmia.

You are to take a targeted history from James (5 years) and his parents (John and Mary) with regard to these episodes of 'loss of consciousness' and formulate a management plan. You are not expected to examine the child.

COMMENTS ON STATION 1

DIAGNOSIS: REPAIR OF AORTIC COARCTATION; TURNER'S SYNDROME

A thorough knowledge of cardiovascular defects, their management and their sequelae is vital for the exam. It is important that you know what the common scars look like – reading about a lateral thoracotomy scar is *not* the same as having seen one. In this case the small secondary scar is probably from a chest drain.

It is important to let the examiner know that you would measure a four-limb BP in addition to plotting the length, weight and head circumference on the appropriate chart. An ECG, CXR and echocardiogram are essential first-line investigations of a significant murmur with no innocent features.

This child has had a repair of aortic coarctation; the pedal oedema is important as it suggests an underlying diagnosis of Turner's syndrome. It is not a feature of cardiac failure in this circumstance. Karyotyping of a blood sample will be diagnostic in the majority of cases.

The clinical features of Turner's syndrome (congenital lymphoedema, short stature and gonadal dysgenesis) can be divided into neonatal, childhood and adolescent findings. You should become familiar with Turner's syndrome as the children are generally well but require prolonged follow-up. Extensive detail is provided here as this same child could be used for the communication skills stations – 'Explain to this child's parents what a diagnosis of Turner's syndrome means?' – or as a history-taking/management-planning scenario.

Age	Clinical findings
Neonatal	Dorsal oedema of hands and feet Redundant nuchal skin folds (secondary to in utero cystic hygromas) Low birth weight and reduced length 17–45% cardiac lesion (bicuspid aortic valve, coarctation of aorta, aortic stenosis, hypoplastic left heart) Developmental dysplasia of the hip (DDH) more common
Childhood	Short stature (proportional) 10% developmental delay Facial abnormalities (epicanthic folds, small mandible, prominent ears, high palate) Webbed neck Low posterior hairline Prominent 'shield' chest Widely spaced nipples Cubitum valgum Hyperconvex fingernails Grommits for 'glue ear' common
Teenage	Failed onset of pubertal development (10% have breast enlargement) Progressively more prominent pigmented naevi 30% renal abnormalities 70% impairment of non-verbal perceptual motor and visuospatial skills 15–30% hypothyroid Scoliosis, lordosis and kyphosis more common

GENETIC ABNORMALITY

Turner's syndrome occurs in 1 in 2500 to 1 in 3000 female live births. The most frequent genetic abnormality is monosomy X (45,X; 50%). The remainder of cases may have a duplication of the long arm of one X (46,X,i(Xq)) or a mosaicism (e.g., 45,X/46,XX). One to two percent of all conceptuses have 45,XO karyotype but over 99% will spontaneously abort.

MANAGEMENT ISSUES

At the time of diagnosis with Turner's syndrome it is important to have baseline investigations: cardiac echocardiogram, thyroid function tests, hearing test, renal ultrasound scan, ovarian function tests, growth assessment and a psychosocial assessment.

Aortic dissection is a significant concern in patients with structural cardiac abnormalities, hypertension or a combination of the two. Hypertension should be treated aggressively. Bacterial endocarditis prophylaxis may be required. Bear this in mind as dental malocclusion is common and may be treated prophylactically. Cardiac disorders in Turner's syndrome are the reason for the increase in mortality in this condition. A nice touch in any discussion with parents is to acknowledge the increased risk of keloid scar formation – important if you are to have a large scar on your chest!

Recombinant human growth hormone (GH) supplementation is offered despite the patients not having a GH deficiency. The supplementation is thought to improve final height. Therapy should be initiated when height is below the fifth centile for age-matched normal females (may be before 2 years of age). Oxandrolone (anabolic steroid) in low dose will also increase final adult height and may be used in conjunction with GH.

Thyroid function should be assessed initially and from the age of 10 years.

Oestrogen therapy from 12–13 years will help the development of secondary sexual characteristics but will not affect final height. In fact, as oestrogen therapy encourages epiphyseal plate closure it may inhibit full height potential.

There is also an increased risk of Crohn's disease (Crohn's is linked to the X chromosome).

CAN YOU ...

Explain to parents that their infant child has been given a diagnosis of Turner's syndrome? What will this mean for their child in the short and long term?

COMMENTS ON STATION 2

DIAGNOSIS: LEUKAEMIA

In this station you have been presented with a Cushingoid 10-year-old with signs of anaemia, petechiae, alopecia and a central venous line.

The most likely reasons for a child having a central venous line are shown in the table below.

Patient	Notes
Oncological	Needs chemotherapy
Haematological	Haemophilia requiring regular Factor VIII injections
Gastrointestinal	Total parenteral nutrition, e.g. short gut syndrome (secondary to Crohn's disease or neonatal enterocolitis)
Renal	Red and blue ends for afferent and efferent lumens for haemodialysis
Immune deficient	Regular antibiotics or immunoglobulin replacement

In this case there is a suggestion of bone marrow failure and enlarged liver and spleen, making the most likely underlying diagnosis malignancy (in particular, leukaemia). The Cushingoid appearances are secondary to the high-dose steroid chemotherapy.

In addition to following the instruction to examine the abdominal system it is important that you demonstrate any lymphoreticular abnormality, so check the cervical, axillary and groin nodes (with permission) for lympha-denopathy. It is also important to decide whether the child is in cardiac failure secondary to the anaemia. You may also see scars on the iliac crests from bone marrow aspirates or at the site of previous lumbar punctures.

Presentation of these findings should be done succinctly; for example:

'This 10-year-old boy has Cushingoid features, alopecia, pallor, petechiae and a central venous catheter in situ. He has no cardiorespiratory compromise. The abdomen is distended and he has hepatosplenomegaly. The liver is palpable three finger-breadths and his spleen is palpable four finger-breadths below the costal margins. There is no evidence of other masses or free abdominal fluid. These findings are consistent with a haematological malignancy such as leukaemia and the consequences of its treatment.

I would like to measure the blood pressure, examine his external genitalia, plot his height and weight on the relevant growth chart and dipstick the urine. My first-line investigations would include a full blood count, blood film and clotting analysis.'

Note that the term 'finger-breadths' was used rather than an estimated span in centimetres; it will save you having to bring out a tape measure when the examiner challenges you! Paediatric oncology is an important subspecialty to which the candidate may not have been exposed; however, it is vital prior to the examination to have sought clinical experience in this area. In the communication skills station you could be required to 'break the bad news' to the parents of a child with newly diagnosed acute lymphoblastic leukaemia, while in the history-taking/management planning scenario you may have to discuss with patients and their families the common problems affecting their chronic care. You must be able to explain the side effects of long-term steroid use; the following mnemonic may help:

Abdominal striae and acne
Buffalo hump
Cataracts
Disability: myopathy and muscle wasting
(o)Edema and osteopenia
Facial changes (moon face)
Growth retardation and glycaemic control
Hypertension and hirsutism
Injury: easy bruising

COMMENTS ON STATION 3

DIAGNOSIS: BENIGN INTRACRANIAL HYPERTENSION

- *What nerve(s) are involved to give this pattern of external ophthalmoplegia?*
  - The left sixth cranial nerve (abducens) is responsible for moving the gaze laterally and is a common isolated cranial nerve palsy.
- *What is the most likely cause of the vomiting?*
  - Raised intracranial pressure is the most important and likely differential diagnosis.
- *What are the causes of the above condition in children?*
  - Raised intracranial pressure has a number of causes. The table below includes the most common.

In this case the child had benign intracranial hypertension (BIH), which may be referred to as a pseudotumour cerebri.

BIH is a condition of idiopathic raised intracranial pressure and, importantly, may lead to papilloedema, progressive optic atrophy and blindness. Its pathogenesis is unclear, but may be due to an increased resistance to the flow of CSF at the arachnoid granulations, thereby reducing the rate of CSF reabsorption. The presenting symptoms may include headaches, tinnitus, diplopia (with sixth nerve palsy) and other visual defects, particularly a 'nasal step' field defect.

The most common risk factors for BIH are endocrine and include female sex, reproductive age group, obesity, hypothalamic–pituitary–adrenal axis disruption, thyroid and parathyroid disorders. The use of certain drugs may be associated with an increased risk of BIH, e.g. corticosteroids, retinoic acid preparations, levothyroxine and tetracycline.

Category	Cause
Intracranial haemorrhage • Extradural haematoma • Subdural haematoma • Subarachnoid haemorrhage • Intracerebral haemorrhage	Traumatic brain injury Expanding arteriovenous malformation Ruptured cerebral artery aneurysm
Infections	Mastoiditis Meningitis Encephalitis
Vascular	Ischaemic infarcts Vasculitis
Neoplastic	Intracranial tumour (primary or metastatic)
Haematology	Sickling syndromes Polycythaemia Prothrombotic states
Other	Hydrocephalus Benign intracranial hypertension Idiopathic

What would be your first-line investigations?

- Bedside tests: blood pressure and urine dipstick analysis.
- Cranial imaging: preferably MRI or CT with contrast to exclude a mass lesion (essential prior to lumbar puncture).
- Formal ophthalmology opinion and visual field testing.
- Lumbar puncture with measurement of opening pressures.
- CSF sent for microscopy, culture, sensitivity, viral studies, glucose and protein.
- Full blood count, sickle cell screen, urea, electrolytes, calcium, coagulation screen and thrombophilia screen.

COMMENTS ON STATION 4

DIAGNOSIS: ASTHMA

If you have helped out in organising a clinical exam you will know that the biggest headache for the senior examiner is making sure all the patients turn up. In most centres one child will have to be replaced at short notice and a well asthmatic on the inpatient ward is the easiest replacement. Common things are common and even the most competent candidate can fall at what should be an easy hurdle. They may have a thorough knowledge of the genetics of Kartagener's syndrome but no appreciation of the latest British Thoracic Society guidelines for asthma!

The differential diagnoses for a child with wheeze (expiratory noise) can be divided as shown in the table below.

System	Conditions
Respiratory: extrathoracic These cause stridor (inspiratory noise) as the predominant symptom	Adenotonsillar hypertrophy Peritonsillar abscess Retropharyngeal abscess Epiglottitis Vocal cord dysfunction
Respiratory: intrathoracic	Tracheal stenosis or web Bacterial tracheitis Tracheo-bronchomalacia Tracheo-oesophageal fistula (H type or repair) Bronchiolitis (in the infant) Vascular ring
Respiratory: functional	Asthma Cystic fibrosis Recurrent aspiration Bronchopulmonary dysplasia (in the ex-pre-term infant) Bronchiectasis (including primary ciliary dyskinesia)
Cardiovascular	Cardiac failure (pulmonary oedema) Cardiomegaly
Gastrointestinal	Gastro-oesophageal reflux
Lymphoreticular	Mediastinal mass/lymphadenopathy Immunodeficiency

What part of the respiratory system examination should you offer to examine next?

It is important to remember to offer to examine the ears, nose and throat in all respiratory cases. You may find nasal polyps, grommets, hearing aids, cleft palate repair or other abnormalities which may assist with the narrowing of your differential. It is also important to remember to palpate for lymphadenopathy.

What additional bedside tests are important in this child?

In asthma and other reactive airways disease it is important to check the child's peak expiratory flow (PEF) or formal spirometry. If there is a PEF meter to hand you may be asked to direct the child yourself, so be sure to be aware of the proper technique. Your hospital should have a children's respiratory nurse. Thirty minutes spent with her will be 30 minutes well spent if you are asked to do this! A knowledge of the variety of asthma devices (inhaler type, spacers, PEF meters) is expected and may be required in almost any of the stations in the exam. Remember that the predicted PEF is proportional to the child's height (approximate PEFR = (height in cm $\times$ 5) – 400).

In addition to the PEF you should ask to see the child's sputum specimen pot (for the thick sticky green secretions seen in cystic fibrosis or bronchiectasis), measure a blood pressure and plot the child's height and weight on the appropriate chart.

REMINDER

- *Harrison's sulcus*: an indentation, of varying severity, in the lower chest caused by chronic airways obstruction
- *Kartagener's syndrome*: the presence of dextrocardia, sinusitis and bronchiectasis with a diagnosis of primary ciliary dyskinesia

COMMENTS ON STATION 5

DIAGNOSIS: NEUROFIBROMATOSIS TYPE 1 (NF1)

Unless you are a lists person try not to compartmentalise your knowledge too much. You will find in the exam that you need to have the ability to think laterally and out of the boxes. However, certain conditions such as Down's, Turner's and the neurocutaneous syndromes lend themselves well to the list approach. Make sure you *know* the list, not *think* you know!

Diagnostic criteria for NF1 include the presence of at least two of the following:

1. *Café au lait* spots:
   - ≥6 over 5 mm if pre-pubertal
   - ≥6 over 15 mm if pubertal
2. Axillary or inguinal freckling
3. Lisch nodules (iris hamartomas) (≥2)
4. Neurofibromas (≥2) or one plexiform neurofibroma
5. Distinctive osseous lesion (kyphoscoliosis, sphenoid wing dysplasia, pseudoarthroses secondary to tibia/fibula bowing)
6. Optic glioma
7. First-degree relative with NF1.

Differential diagnoses for conditions with *café au lait* patches include:

- Tuberous sclerosis
- McCune–Albright syndrome
- Russell–Silver syndrome
- DNA repair disorders:
  - Ataxia telangiectasia
  - Bloom syndrome
  - Fanconi anaemia
- Noonan's syndrome
- Idiopathic.

What systems will you now examine and how will you structure your examination?

Practise answering this question before the exam. It is actually quite difficult to do ad hoc and you may find yourself jumping all over the place. It is important to try and be systematic and it may be more fluid to explain yourself as you go along.

- *Skin*: Examine all skin areas, including the axillae, groin and back.
  - *Findings*: Plexiform neuromas, neurofibromas, pigmented and depigmented patches.
- *Cardiovascular*: Full cardiovascular examination including blood pressure measurement, listening for renal artery bruits and palpating pulses.
  - *Findings*: Renal artery stenosis, hypertension from phaeochromocytoma or coarctation of the aorta; murmur from pulmonary stenosis.
- *Neurological*: Full neurological examination (including peripheral and cranial nerves, cognitive function and head circumference measurement).
  - *Findings*: Macrocephaly, learning difficulties, seizure disorder, localised neuropathy or weakness.
- *Eyes*: Acuity, iris visualisation and fundoscopy.
  - *Findings*: Lisch nodules, optic glioma, hypertensive retinopathy.
- *Musculoskeletal*: Spine and limb examination, standing and sitting height.
  - *Findings*: Scoliosis, pseudoarthrosis (in particular tibial), short stature.
- *Others*: Examine for scars.
  - *Findings*: Malignancy resection especially cranial and spinal tumours (overlap with NF2 with acoustic schwannomas).

Try and decide on a structured examination that allows the incorporation of the different systems. Practise the scheme on patients or colleagues to get used to the task.

The disorder is inherited in an autosomal dominant pattern. Fifty percent are familial and the remainder are new mutations. The disorder has an incidence of approximately 1 in 3000 live births.

Neurofibromin is the protein encoded by the NF1 gene, located at 17q11.2. It encodes a large protein that is expressed in brain, kidney, spleen and thymus tissue.

COMMENTS ON STATION 6

DIAGNOSIS: GLOBAL DEVELOPMENTAL DELAY

The child in this case is actually 15 months old. She has developmental delay with truncal hypotonia. It is important not to make statements regarding the child's true age if it is not known; instead refer to the developmental age.

It is useful to have memorised important milestones – these can be taken from standard texts or assessment tools (e.g. the Denver chart). If you can identify the most advanced task achieved in one developmental area and then demonstrate that the next task is failed it is possible to give a developmental age range. Remember there may be dissociation of development, i.e. one field is more delayed than a second. The developmental age of the child is 6–8 weeks for gross motor but 10 months for fine motor. Both are delayed but discordant with each other.

What additional developmental reflexes could you describe or test in this child?

- *Stepping reflex*: With the child held in the vertical position their feet should be placed on the floor and then lifted lightly. This should encourage the child to make small stepping motions. This is slightly different from the placing reflex, where the feet are moved towards a small raised object. The feet should lift up to stand on that object. Both these reflexes are present at birth and disappear at approximately 6 weeks.
- *Parachute reflex*: The infant is moved rapidly face downwards towards a surface from a prone position. Both arms should spread out to break the fall. It appears at about 6 months but should definitely be present by 12 months. You support the child through the movement and don't let go!
- *Atonic neck reflex*: The child must be supine and the head rotated to either side. The limbs on the side towards which the head is turned should both extend (with flexion of the contralateral limb). This reflex should disappear by 6 months.

This child had an as yet undiagnosed central neurological problem. Interestingly, her fine motor skills are more developed than her gross motor skills. Do not let this put you off. The developmental station is testing your assessment skills as a paediatrician, not your diagnostic skills as a geneticist or a neurologist.

However, it is important to assess developmental areas individually and not assume an obviously disabled child is delayed in all areas.

COMMENTS ON STATION 7

This is bread-and-butter paediatrics and your examiner would expect you to perform to a high standard in order to pass the station. In order to do this you will need to have an understanding of asthma management in both acute and outpatient settings. Obviously, you must understand the advantages and disadvantages of interventions such as inhaled steroid. Also you must predict what the mother's agenda is likely to be. What was the reason she didn't want to start preventative treatment? This is a communication station so a regurgitation of facts about the British Thoracic Society (BTS) guidelines will be of no use if mum is concerned because her mother fractured her hip secondary to steroid use!

How would you initiate the conversation?

On entering the room you should take on the role assigned (in this case the registrar) and introduce yourself as Dr X. You should confirm their names and then politely thank them for coming to see you and explain that you hope not to be disturbed through the consultation. It is good practice early on to let them know that they should feel free to interrupt you and ask questions if anything is unclear.

What do you expect the mother will want to know about the inhaled steroid?

The key to this station is listening attentively and finding out any specific concerns. This is, after all, a communication skills station and you will be expected to show active listening skills. You should then address concerns appropriately.

It is likely that the mother will have heard about steroids and the possible side effects. Often in communication stations a family member has previously been affected deleteriously by a particular drug and the family have obvious concerns for their child being given that drug.

System	Side effects
Skin	Skin thinning, purpura, alopecia, striae, 'Cushingoid facies'
Eye	Cataracts, glaucoma
Cardiovascular	Hypertension, hyperlipidaemia
Gastrointestinal	Gastritis and ulceration, pancreatitis, bowel perforation
Renal	Fluid and electrolyte imbalance
Musculoskeletal	Myopathy, osteoporosis, avascular necrosis
Neurological	Hyperactivity, benign intracranial hypertension, euphoria
Endocrine	Diabetes mellitus, secondary adrenal insufficiency
Immune system	Increased opportunistic and standard infections

In this case you will be able to reassure her that inhaled steroids at the standard dosing do not have the side effects seen in systemic corticosteroid therapy. Inhaled corticosteroids have been shown to cause oral candidiasis; there are case reports of adrenal suppression and short-term linear growth restriction but with attainment of normal adult height.

The inhaled corticosteroids reduce symptoms and improve lung function, while uncontrolled asthma has the potential to cause significant growth restriction, impair exercise tolerance and has an associated mortality. The inhaled steroid dosing should be reviewed regularly and the dose gradually reduced to the lowest that provides good symptom control.

What would you include in an asthma plan for an acute exacerbation?

The BTS again provide up-to-date guidance on this issue. A written asthma plan should be provided for every patient and may be divided into:

1. Mild/intermittent symptoms:
   - Take regular prevention medication as prescribed.
   - Use reliever inhaler (e.g. two puffs salbutamol every 4 hours) as required.
2. Moderate symptoms:
   - Take regular prevention medication as prescribed.
   - Start oral prednisolone if prescribed by your doctor.
   - Use reliever inhaler (e.g. 2–10 puffs salbutamol every 3–4 hours).
   - Seek medical help within 24–36 hours if no improvement in symptoms.
3. Severe symptoms (e.g. too breathless to talk):
   - Use reliever inhaler (e.g.10 puffs salbutamol). If no improvement after 5 minutes call for an ambulance and repeat reliever every 20 minutes.

What would be the key issues for managing and monitoring background symptoms?

There is clear guidance from the BTS on the management of asthma. You should ensure that you have read and understood the latest edition of the guidelines (*www.brit-thoracic.org.uk*).

The management of asthma should include the following:

- Minimise aggravating factors (e.g. smoking).
- Maximise patient concordance with treatment (e.g. by patient education).
- Patient-oriented goals.
- Age-appropriate treatment delivery (e.g. spacer device with mask for infants).
- Appropriate medication (as per 'stepwise policy').
- Appropriate referral to specialist care.
- Aim for minimal symptoms, minimise exacerbations, minimal intervention and normality of life.

This is a common scenario in life as a neonatal registrar, in interviews and exams. Remember that the station is targeted at assessing your communication skills and understanding of ethics rather than your in-depth understanding of neonatology.

As with all cases, it is essential to start with a clear introduction of your name and position. You should ask the couple their preferred names and remember to use them in the interview. It would look good if you told the couple that you had made arrangements not to be disturbed. You should ask the couple if they know if the baby is a boy or girl or if they have decided upon a name (so you don't have to refer to the baby as 'it'!).

What does resuscitation of a 24-week gestation newborn involve?

For this communication skills station it is useful to have worked on the neonatal unit and to have been involved in the resuscitation of extremely premature babies. For aspects of newborn life support (NLS) you should refer to the Resuscitation Council (*www.resus.org.uk*) course material. The following is a simple outline of the proceedings:

1. Experienced neonatal team in attendance at the delivery.
2. Neonatal 'Resuscitaire', equipment and drugs should be available.
3. Once the baby is born it is transferred to the Resuscitaire to be kept warm and to allow an initial assessment to be made (tone, colour, respiration, heart rate, response and, in the case of extreme prematurity, viability).
4. The baby is then intubated (prophylactic surfactant may be given), ventilation initiated and cardiac massage given with drug administration if appropriate.
5. The baby is transferred to the neonatal unit when stabilised.

An initial approach to the subject might be to ask the couple what they thought would happen if their baby were to be born prematurely. You may find they know far more than you expected or much less than you'd hoped! You can then tailor your discussion to suit their understanding.

In this scenario the following important points may be mentioned:

1. *'It is sadly not possible for all babies born at this gestation to survive, and the initial resuscitation and first 24 hours are the most crucial.'*
2. *'The resuscitation of an extremely pre-term baby will involve a lot of people and the baby will require a tube being placed into its windpipe for us to give some medicine and to help him or her breathe.'*
3. *'If we are able to stabilise your baby we will take him/her to the neonatal unit where we will keep the baby warm, give fluids by drip and necessary medications.'*
4. *'Babies born this prematurely are poorly developed, in particularly the lungs and brain, and it is possible that the baby will have some long-term problems because of this fact.'*

In the UK, morbidity and mortality data are available for neonates born prematurely through the Epicure study (*bmj.bmjjournals.com/cgi/content/full/319/7217/1093/DC1*).

Don't be afraid to offer meetings, patient information sheets or follow-up appointments in the scenarios – if it is available in a hospital it can be 'available' here too.

The couple may ask you not to resuscitate the baby when it is born. In this situation you must be sure of your legal and ethical responsibility. It would be important to offer the couple an urgent meeting with the duty consultant. The Royal College of Paediatrics and Child Health (UK) provide guidance in the publication *Withholding and Withdrawing Life Sustaining Treatment in Children: A Framework for Practice*, May 2004.

Within the document there is a discussion of five occasions when it may be ethical and legal to consider withholding treatment (see p. 119):

1. The 'brain dead' child
2. The 'permanent vegetative state'
3. The 'no chance' situation
4. The 'no purpose' situation
5. The 'unbearable' situation.

Should there be a precipitous delivery prior to resolution of this issue, there is a responsibility to offer resuscitation to an infant showing signs of life.

COMMENTS ON STATION 9

This station is designed to assess your communication skills with the family and history-taking ability. You should follow the instructions given and focus your history on the presenting complaint for the majority of the time. Your time management in this station is essential, and remember: you can always finish talking with the family a minute early and collect your thoughts prior to presenting to the examiner.

How will you structure the interview?

In the time you have available outside the station you should decide what areas you want to cover in the history. A structure for the interview may then be as follows:

1. Initial introduction and clarification of reason for attending the clinic.
2. Period of active listening to ensure you have given the family a chance to tell you their concerns.
3. Directed questioning to ensure you have investigated your differential diagnoses appropriately with a detailed history of a typical 'attack'.
   - When did the first one happen?
   - What was he doing beforehand?
   - Where were you when it started?
   - What was the first thing you noticed?
   - What happened next?

4. Repeat the main concerns back to the family and give them another opportunity to add to or clarify them for you.
5. Complete a systematic history. You may want to particularly expand upon the social, schooling and family history.

At the end you should have a good idea of what happened, the main problems, any associated features/precipitants/family history and the nature of these problems, and have formulated a plan of action.

What are your differential diagnoses for 'loss of consciousness' in this age group?

System	Cause
Neurological	Seizure disorder Behavioural Reflex anoxic seizure Cerebrovascular accident
Respiratory	Respiratory arrest with hypoxia Cough syncope Breath-holding
Cardiovascular	Tachyarrhythmias (SVT, long Q–T) Bradyarrhythmias (AV conduction defects) Cardiomyopathy Vasovagal episodes Postural hypotension Shock, including anaphylaxis Left ventricular outflow obstruction, including aortic stenosis Congenital heart disease (including Fallot's tetralogy) Pulmonary hypertension
Metabolic	Hypoglycaemia
Drug-induced	Inhaled nitrites Antihypertensive agents Tricyclic antidepressant Drugs of abuse (unlikely intentional at this age)

What will your management plan involve?

The plan will depend on the likely cause and this will be determined by information gained in the history. It is known that most children will have normal investigations following a loss of consciousness.

For recurrent episodes that you feel are likely cardiac in origin you may suggest:

- 12-lead ECG and/or exercise testing
- Echocardiography
- Holter monitor (24-hour ambulatory ECG recording)

- Tilt table testing
- Full blood count.

If you feel that the episodes are representing seizure activity, you could suggest:

- Event diary
- Electroencephalogram
- Neuroimaging (CT/MRI)
- Blood glucose, urea and electrolytes, liver function tests, calcium and magnesium.

It is important to give a clear management plan, but do not be ashamed of including in the plan that you would discuss the case with your consultant. It is better to be cautious and ask for advice from senior colleagues.

Circuit H

STATION 1

This station assesses your ability to elicit clinical signs:
- **CVS**

This is a 9-minute station of clinical interaction. You will have up to 4 minutes beforehand to prepare yourself. No additional information will be given or is necessary before commencing the station. When the bell sounds you will be invited into the examination room.

INTRODUCTION

On entering the room you are asked to examine a 4-month-old infant who has been referred to you because a murmur was heard at a routine health check.

CLINICAL SCENARIO

The infant looks small for his age but is pink and well perfused. You ask the mother to undress the child carefully and then perform a full cardiovascular examination.

The child lacks substantial muscle bulk but you find good peripheral pulses, heart rate of 140/min, with no cyanosis. The child's respiratory rate is 50. There are no scars on the chest, and the mediastinum is not displaced. A long systolic murmur is heard loudest at the lower left sternal edge and radiates throughout the precordium but not to the back. There is a palpable thrill at the lower left sternal edge but no heave.

What further examination features would you wish to elicit at this point?

What additional information would you request at the end of the examination?

What investigation would you primarily request and what lesion do you expect to find?

STATION 2

This station assesses your ability to elicit clinical signs:
- **Abdo/Other**

This is a 9-minute station of clinical interaction. You will have up to 4 minutes beforehand to prepare yourself. No additional information will be given or is necessary before commencing the station. When the bell sounds you will be invited into the examination room.

INTRODUCTION

On entering the room you are asked to perform an abdominal examination on the 1-month-old child who recently presented to a paediatric ambulatory clinic.

CLINICAL SCENARIO

The infant is alert and active. It is clear from initial inspection that the child is jaundiced. There are no peripheral stigmata of abdominal disease. The pulse is 130/min and the CRT is less than 2 seconds. The infant has yellow sclera and has no pallor. The respiration is comfortable and there are no scars or skin abnormalities visible on the chest.

The abdomen is distended asymmetrically, with the right side more prominent. There are no scars or distended veins. The abdomen is soft and non-tender. You find a palpable liver three finger-breadths below the right costal margin. There is no other organomegaly or masses. Bowel sounds are present. There are normal male genitalia. There is no lymphadenopathy. A dirty nappy is next to the patient.

What is the most important diagnosis to exclude?

What further information do you request to supplement your examination?

What would your first-line investigations include?

STATION 3

This station assesses your ability to elicit clinical signs:
- **Neurological**

This is a 9-minute station of clinical interaction. You will have up to 4 minutes beforehand to prepare yourself. No additional information will be given or is necessary before commencing the station. When the bell sounds you will be invited into the examination room.

INTRODUCTION

You are asked to assess the gait of a 10-year-old girl.

CLINICAL SCENARIO

The girl is sitting down next to her mother. She looks well and is the appropriate size for her age. She tells you she is able to walk without assistance. She has her lower limbs sufficiently exposed and is able to get up from the chair without any problem. There is no obvious wasting or deformity to her legs. You ask her to walk to the end of the room and then to walk back. No abnormality is apparent. You ask her to walk on her tiptoes, on the sides of her feet and on her heels, all of which she is able to begin to do but with difficulty. She stumbles on a few occasions. You ask her to stand upright, feet together, and find she is stable; however, when Romberg's test is performed it is found to be positive.

The examiner asks you what you would like to examine next.

You move on to examine her lower limb neurology. Tone and power in both legs are normal. You elicit knee jerks but have great difficulty in obtaining an ankle reflex response. You are not sure whether this is your technique or a positive clinical sign. You continue on to examine sensation, which appears intact. Joint position sense, however, appears to be absent bilaterally in the big toes and ankles. You suddenly remember you haven't examined coordination or the plantar response but the examiner stops you due to time restraint.

How would you present your findings and what additional information would you request from the examiner to supplement the examination?

What would you expect to find on testing vibration?

You are not asked for a diagnosis, but what would you be considering?

This station assesses your ability to elicit clinical signs:

- **Respiratory/Other**

This is a 9-minute station of clinical interaction. You will have up to 4 minutes beforehand to prepare yourself. No additional information will be given or is necessary before commencing the station. When the bell sounds you will be invited into the examination room.

INTRODUCTION

The examiner asks you to examine a 5-year-old child who presented to the ward with a cough.

CLINICAL SCENARIO

The child looks well, with no sign of respiratory distress. He is not requiring oxygen and can respond to questions in full sentences.

You note on general inspection that he has bilateral hearing aids, has a vertical linear scar in his top lip and has a portacath on the left side of the chest. You enter into your routine respiratory examination and find that he is clubbed but has no peripheral or central cyanosis. His pulse is 100/min and his respiratory rate is 25/min. He has no other external facial abnormalities and on oral examination you note that the hard and soft palate are also scarred.

On chest inspection you note the portacath on the left and a healed scar on the right side from a presumed previous port. There are no other scars. The chest expands equally and has a resonant percussion note throughout. There are coarse diffuse breath sounds bilaterally on auscultation but no focal crepitations or bronchial breathing. You examine for a liver edge and it is not palpable.

What clinical sign may be present on deeper examination of the mouth?

How will you present this information to the examiner?

What further aspects of the clinical examination are required?

What additional bedside tests would you perform?

Can you demonstrate to the examiner how to check for clubbing?

STATION 5

This station assesses your ability to elicit clinical signs:

- **Other**

This is a 9-minute station of clinical interaction. You will have up to 4 minutes beforehand to prepare yourself. No additional information will be given or is necessary before commencing the station. When the bell sounds you will be invited into the examination room.

INTRODUCTION

On entering the room the examiner instructs you to examine a system of your choice in the child in front of you.

A school-age Caucasian boy is seated next to his mother. He is wearing glasses. You note that he has a marked pearly pink acneiform rash over his nose and cheeks.

What is your first thought in terms of a diagnosis?

CLINICAL SCENARIO

You inform the examiner that you would like to examine his skin for other lesions associated with the condition.

In his hands you note periungual fibromas on a couple of his fingers. The chest reveals a number of smooth-bordered hypomelanotic patches. You also note a number of pigmented *café au lait* patches.

The examiner agrees with your findings and asks if you would like to examine any other systems. What physical findings would you wish to elicit to show your understanding of the condition?

The examiner asks you if there are any questions you wish to ask the mother. How would you respond and what would you ask?

This station assesses your ability to assess specifically requested areas in a child with a developmental problem:

- **Development**

This is a 9-minute station of clinical interaction. You will have up to 4 minutes beforehand to prepare yourself. No additional information will be given or is necessary before commencing the station. When the bell sounds you will be invited into the examination room.

INTRODUCTION

You are instructed to talk the examiner through your developmental assessment of this 3-year-old girl. The child is accompanied by her mother and you note that she is in a pushchair with specific modifications for positional support. You make the following observations:

- *Gross motor*: You see spontaneous movements of all four limbs but with apparent spasticity bilaterally. She has poor head control. You ask her mother regarding her ability to roll, sit or stand and find that she will do none of them.
- *Fine motor and vision*: She does not reach for objects. She will hold toys placed in her hand but does not transfer them. There is no demonstrable pincer grip, though she has lost the grasp reflex. You note that she has bilateral coloboma of the iris. You test her ability to fix on your face and follow it to 90 or 180°. You do the same with a red toy and in both situations note that she is unable to follow. She appears to have a wandering gaze.
- *Speech, language and hearing*: You ask if the child has any language – noises, coos, babbles, words. The mother explains that she simply makes screams or non-specific noise. You ask if the child has had a hearing test and whether she seems to respond to noises by startling or quietening to her mother's voice.

What tests do you know for hearing and vision at different ages that may be appropriate for a child with this level of developmental delay?

- *Social, emotional and behaviour*: You are unable to elicit any smiles or laughter and ask the mother if there have been any such actions noted by her. You note that the child is still in a nappy. The mother tells you she is fed orally but is fully dependent for toileting, though will cry when 'dirty'.

What is the developmental age of this child in each of the areas of development?

STATION 7

This station assesses your ability to communicate appropriate, factually correct information in an effective way within the emotional context of the clinical setting:

- **Communication One**

This is a 9-minute station consisting of spoken interaction. You will have up to 2 minutes before the start of the station to read this sheet and prepare yourself. You may make notes on the paper provided.

When the bell sounds you will be invited into the examination room. Please take this instruction sheet with you. The examiner will not ask questions during the 9 minutes but will warn you when you have approximately 2 minutes left.

You are not required to examine a patient.

The encounter should be focused on the task; you will be penalised for asking irrelevant questions or providing superfluous information. You will be marked on your ability to communicate, not the speed with which you convey information. You may not have time to complete the communication.

SETTING

You are the SpR on the neonatal unit.

SCENARIO

You are to inform the mother of James that he has had two surface swabs positive for MRSA which were taken on his arrival at your unit. You should advise her of the management plan. James is to be nursed in isolation and receive topical treatment for the MRSA. He was previously in an SCBU bay with five other babies.

BACKGROUND INFORMATION

James was born at 38/40 gestation by elective LSCS with a birth weight of 3.7 kg. He is his mother's first baby. At the 20/40 antenatal scan he was found to have gastroschisis. He was delivered at the tertiary centre and operated on shortly after birth. He has recovered well and was transferred over to your hospital (his local DGH) for establishment of breast-feeding on day 14. His scar is healing well and he is now on full enteral feeds. He is still awaiting the results of his chromosome analysis.

His mother is a 34-year-old history teacher.

How will you introduce the topic of MRSA?

If the mother reacts aggressively, how will you calm her?

The mother has heard of the 'killer bug'. How do you address this?

STATION 8

This station assesses your ability to communicate appropriate, factually correct information in an effective way within the emotional context of the clinical setting:

- **Communication Two**

This is a 9-minute station consisting of spoken interaction. You will have up to 2 minutes before the start of the station to read this sheet and prepare yourself. You may make notes on the paper provided.

When the bell sounds you will be invited into the examination room. Please take this instruction sheet with you. The examiner will not ask questions during the 9 minutes but will warn you when you have approximately 2 minutes left.

You are not required to examine a patient.

The encounter should be focused on the task; you will be penalised for asking irrelevant questions or providing superfluous information. You will be marked on your ability to communicate, not the speed with which you convey information. You may not have time to complete the communication.

SETTING

You are the SpR in the general paediatric outpatient clinic.

SCENARIO

You are to give the results of the investigations, formulate a management plan and convey this to David's mother.

BACKGROUND INFORMATION

David is 19 months old. He was seen 4 weeks ago in the paediatric admissions unit. He had presented with a history of tasting a small amount of peanut butter and within 10 minutes having developed a blotchy, raised erythematous itchy reaction over his whole body. He had become wheezy at this time, though this resolved with no specific treatment. He received paracetamol only.

His subsequent examination and developmental assessment were normal.

He has a family history of atopy, with his father suffering from asthma and his mother suffering from hay fever.

He had the following investigations:

- RAST to peanut 200 IU (negative to other nuts and milk)
- Skin test to peanut ++++ (negative to other nuts and milk).

What management plan would you recommend and would you prescribe the adrenaline (epinephrine) pen device (EpiPen)?

What additional follow-up would you arrange?

How could you check that the mother has understood your instructions?

This station assesses your ability to take a focused history and explain to the parent your diagnosis or differential management plan.

- History-taking and Management planning

This is a 22-minute station of spoken interaction. You will have up to 4 minutes beforehand to prepare yourself. The scenario is below. Be aware that you should focus on the task given. You will be penalised for asking irrelevant questions or providing superfluous information. When the bell sounds you will be invited into the examination room. You will have 13 minutes with the patient (with a warning when you have 4 minutes left). You will then have a short period to reflect on the case while the patient leaves the room. You will then have 9 minutes with the examiner.

SETTING

You are the SpR in the general paediatric outpatient department.

SCENARIO

You are to see Clare, an 8-year-old girl with Rett's syndrome.

Your task is to take a focused history regarding Clare's diet and recent problem of poor weight gain and formulate a management plan.

You are not expected to examine Clare.

BACKGROUND INFORMATION

Clare was diagnosed with Rett's syndrome at age 3 years. She has developmental delay, feeding difficulties and has recently had a gastrostomy sited. Her weight has been static and she has been more tired recently. Her current weight is 18.3 kg.

COMMENTS ON STATION 1

DIAGNOSIS: VENTRICULAR SEPTAL DEFECT REQUIRING MEDICAL/SURGICAL INTERVENTION

It is important when performing the cardiovascular exam to be thinking of what your findings imply as you go. The fact that the child is pink suggests that there is an acyanotic cardiac lesion. However, the evidence of poor growth and distress indicates the lesion is compromising. This child has a ventricular septal defect and must be examined for signs of failure. In this case it would be important to examine the abdomen for a palpable liver edge (and if present decide if it is pulsatile/smooth and determine the liver span by percussion) and then check that the femoral pulses are present. As the child has a thrill the murmur must be at least grade 4.

This child will need referral to a paediatric cardiologist for input in regard to diuretics, ACE inhibitors and surgical closure of the defect. Do not forget to comment on the child's nutritional status – feeding will be an issue and the child will need calorie supplementation and potentially nasogastric feeds.

At the end of all cardiological examinations it is useful to state what you would go on to do and be prepared to do it. The following are general but not specific:

1. Measure the blood pressure.
2. Plot the weight, length and head circumference on the appropriate chart.
3. Dipstick the urine (for haematuria associated with endocarditis).

An ECG would be useful in determining any electrical abnormality and may help narrow the differentials. You should by now have a well-structured approach to the childhood ECG. It may be complicated by age, congenital heart defects and conduction defects, but a few simple steps can help you locate the abnormalities and look for evidence of developing complications. The two key features to comment on are:

- Axis:
  - Right   Right ventricular hypertrophy
    ASD (ostium secundum), also look for RSR in V1
    Hypoplastic left heart
  - Left   Left ventricular hypertrophy
    Partial AVSD (ostium primum) with RSR in V1
    Cardiac pacing
  - Superior   Complete AVSD (think Down's)
- Voltage criteria:
  - Right hypertrophy   Pulmonary stenosis
    ASD
    Cor pulmonale
    Eisenmenger's reaction
  - Left   VSD or AVSD
    Aortic coarctation or stenosis
    Hypertension.

A chest radiograph may be helpful in the diagnosis of congenital heart disease, and may be performed along with an ECG in hospitals with limited availability of echocardiography. The X-ray film should be analysed for:

1. Heart size and cardiothymic silhouette.
2. Size and prominence of the specific cardiac chambers and great arteries.
3. Pulmonary vascular markings and pulmonary plethora/oligaemia.
4. Associated abnormalities in bones/lungs/abdominal viscera (e.g. situs inversus, midline liver in asplenia/polysplenia, rib notching in older child with coarctation of the aorta, absent thymus in Di George).

Classical appearances in congenital heart defects include:

1. The 'boot-shaped heart' with oligaemic lung fields seen in cyanotic tetralogy of Fallot or some children with tricuspid atresia.
2. The 'egg-shaped heart' with plethoric lung fields and narrow pedicle in the cyanotic infant with transposition of the great arteries.
3. The 'snowman in a snowdrift' with plethoric lung fields and dilated SVC seen in supracardiac type of total anomalous pulmonary venous drainage (TAPVD).

COMMENTS ON STATION 2

DIAGNOSIS: BILIARY ATRESIA

The most important diagnosis to exclude in this child is biliary atresia, a condition with incidence 1 in 10 000 to 1 in 20 000 births, characterised by inflammation and subsequent obliteration of the extrahepatic biliary tract. This process may begin in utero and the pathological stimulus is still unknown. The definitive diagnosis is usually made by liver biopsy; however, information from liver ultrasound scan, duodenal aspirate analysis, endoscopic retrograde cholangiopancreatography (ERCP) or hepatobiliary scintigraphy may indicate the diagnosis.

It is particularly important to make the diagnosis by 2 months of age as the success of the operative treatment (Kasai procedure or hepatoportoenterostomy) is significantly reduced after this time. This procedure enables the infant to grow and improve in nutritional state, and allows the definitive treatment of liver transplantation to be delayed. Without treatment hepatic failure will develop, with marked pruritus being a common problem in the late presenters (treat with cholestyramine). Regardless of whether a Kasai procedure is performed or not it is vital to ensure good growth and nutrition.

In the case of a jaundiced baby, your differentials will be guided by the age of the child and the clinical findings:

- A breast-fed child less that 3 weeks old with a 'yellow' jaundice, normal stool and no other clinical finding is likely to have 'breast milk jaundice'.
- A 2-month-old with mild 'green' jaundice, hepatomegaly, and a right hypochondrial incision may be post-Kasai procedure for biliary atresia.

- A 4-month-old with 'green' jaundice plus hepatomegaly, a central abdominal scar, abnormal umbilicus and a central line may well have TPN-induced conjugated jaundice (following surgery for neonatal necrotising enterocolitis or gastroschisis repair).

At the end of the examination in this case it is important to ask for the following:

1. Check the colour of the stool – grey is bad!
2. Urine sample dipstick for evidence of infection, reducing substances (as found in galactosaemia), and bilirubin.
3. Plotted weight, head circumference and length on the appropriate chart.
4. Blood pressure.

The management of an infant with prolonged jaundice is one of the most common scenarios faced by paediatricians all over the world. There are many causes of jaundice in this age group, lists of which can be found in any paediatric textbook, and as such a structure to the history, examination and investigation is paramount.

History	Gestation at birth Birth trauma/cephalohaematoma Method of feeding Parenteral nutrition Significant family history Maternal and infant blood group Colour of urine and stool
Examination	Dehydration Dysmorphism, e.g. Alagille's Bruising Pruritus Hepatomegaly Other features of note Inspect stool (e.g. pale stools and dark urine)
Initial investigation	Full blood count and reticulocytes Blood film Group and Coombs' Packed cell volume Total and conjugated bilirubin Liver function test Urine: microscopy and culture Urinary bilirubin
Further tests	G6PD assay Urine metabolic screen Thyroid function TORCH Hepatic serology

Investigating conjugated hyperbilirubinaemia (function)	Clotting Blood sugar
Investigating conjugated hyperbilirubinaemia (diagnosis)	Liver ultrasound HIDA scan Liver biopsy α_1-Antitrypsin Detailed endocrine investigation Bilirubin transport/conjugation defects Detailed metabolic investigation

One would usually investigate a jaundiced infant at 2 weeks (if term and formula fed), 3 weeks (if pre-term or breast-fed) or as a matter of urgency if there is a history of jaundice accompanied by pale/grey/acholic stools and dark urine or the infant is systemically unwell (e.g. possible sepsis).

COMMENTS ON STATION 3

DIAGNOSIS: FRIEDREICH'S ATAXIA

This 10-year-old girl looks well but has some subtle signs of instability of her gait and has definite sensory ataxia (positive Romberg's). The joint position sense was abnormal at both great toes. This pattern of abnormality is consistent with posterior column spinal cord dysfunction.

As well as remembering to examine coordination it would be useful to examine her vibration sense and two-point discrimination as these are also carried by fibres in the posterior columns.

Romberg's test is designed to detect the inability of a patient to maintain a steady standing position with one's feet together and eyes closed. You should position the patient standing on a flat surface. You may give the patient a gentle nudge to see if they are able to compensate and maintain their balance. You should always be nearby to catch them should they start to fall. A positive Romberg's test suggests a vestibular dysfunction, cerebellar ataxia or a proprioceptive dysfunction.

Posterior column degeneration in the spinal cord is a feature of Friedreich's ataxia.

Friedreich's ataxia is an autosomal recessive degenerative neurological condition. It is one of the most common inherited ataxias, occurring in 1 in 50000 Caucasians. For those interested, the genetic abnormality is usually a homozygous expansion of the trinucleotide repeat (GAA) sequence in intron 1 of the frataxin gene (chromosome 9q13). The instability caused by these trinucleotide expansions leads to a reduced production of the gene product, a mitochondrial protein called frataxin, thought to have a role in the regulation of iron metabolism.

The major clinical manifestations of Friedreich's ataxia are progressive neurological dysfunction, cardiomyopathy and diabetes mellitus. The disease presentation is variable but early loss of joint position sense and vibration sense is typical. There is preservation of pain and temperature sensation. A progressive ataxia of all four limbs and gait occurs as a result of cerebellar dysfunction, often by 15 years of age.

The following pattern may be seen on examination:

- Cerebellar ataxia, dysarthria and nystagmus
- Wheelchair use (mean age of onset 11–25 years)
- Romberg's test is positive
- Deep tendon reflexes are absent
- Plantar response is extensor due to pyramidal tract disease
- Pain/temperature sensation preserved
- Distal muscle atrophy (hands and feet)
- Intelligence preserved
- Skeletal abnormalities (pes cavus, hammer toes and progressive kyphoscoliosis)
- Visual impairment (due to optic atrophy) and swallow dysfunction
- Hypertrophic cardiomyopathy and arrhythmias.

There is no established treatment for Friedreich's ataxia but a multidisciplinary team approach is essential. Antioxidant mechanisms and supplementation (idebenone, coenzyme Q10 and vitamin E) are under investigation as treatment options.

REMINDER

The mnemonic DANISH is used to look for signs of cerebellar dysfunction:

Dysdiadochokinesia
Ataxia
Nystagmus
Intention tremor
Slurred speech
Hyporeflexia

COMMENTS ON STATION 4

DIAGNOSIS: BRONCHIECTASIS; CLEFT LIP AND PALATE; HEARING IMPAIRMENT

A cleft palate (with or without cleft lip) is a common finding, with an incidence of 1 in 1000 live births. If you perform a deeper oral examination of this child's mouth you may find a bifid uvula, an abnormality present in 1 in 80 patients with cleft palate. A speech assessment may show nasal speech or evidence of delay due to the associated deafness.

It will be useful to practise giving yourself complicated findings to present to a colleague so that your ability to be precise and confident is improved. In this case it would be advisable to go along the following lines:

'This 5-year-old boy looks comfortable at rest. I note he has bilateral hearing aids and previous facial surgery consistent with a repair of a congenital cleft lip and palate. He is clubbed in his fingers, consistent with chronic respiratory

disease, and on examination of his chest I note that he has a portacath in situ on the left side and a scar in a similar position on the right side. He has diffuse, coarse breath sounds but no evidence of focal consolidation or effusion. The liver is not enlarged or displaced. My primary differential diagnosis is of bronchiectasis with associated bilateral conductive hearing impairment and a repaired cleft palate and lip.'

In a child with bronchiectasis and hearing impairment it would be important to ensure the heart sounds are auscultated and apex position checked for dextrocardia, as is found in 50% of cases of primary ciliary dyskinesia. The liver may be found on the left side in situs inversus.

The standard bedside tests for the respiratory system should include the following:

1. Plot the height, weight and head circumference on the appropriate chart.
2. Peak flow measurement or pulmonary function testing.
3. Ear, nose and throat examination.
4. Sputum sample inspection.

In the case presented it would be important to check the observation chart for pyrexia suggesting an infective exacerbation.

Clubbing is a core respiratory sign (but be aware of the non-respiratory causes too) and it is essential you can clearly demonstrate it to the examiner. One should initially view the finger from the side and observe any excess convex curvature. The nail-bed should be tested for fluctuance and then the nail-bed angle checked by placing the nails of both index fingers together.

REMINDER

Underlying causes of bronchiectasis

Mechanism	Causes
Respiratory	Bronchiolitis obliterans Severe asthma Previous severe pneumonia Pertussis
Genetic	Cystic fibrosis α_1-Antitrypsin deficiency Primary ciliary dyskinesia (autosomal recessive)
Mechanical	Previous inhaled foreign body H-type tracheo-oesophageal fistula
Immune deficiency	Hypogammaglobulinaemia IgA deficiency
Idiopathic	

COMMENTS ON STATION 5

DIAGNOSIS: TUBEROUS SCLEROSIS

The finding of adenoma sebaceum (angiofibromas) as described would make you consider the diagnosis of tuberous sclerosis.

Tuberous sclerosis is a multi-system neurocutaneous disorder associated with a predisposition to benign tumours, most commonly in brain, skin and kidneys. It is an autosomal dominant condition, with an incidence of 1 in 5000 to 1 in 10 000 live births.

In this dominant condition one-third of cases are familial and the remainder (non-familial) are due to spontaneous germ line mutations or mosaicism. There is full penetrance of the condition, but marked variability of phenotypic expression even among affected individuals within the same family.

In the case described it would be important to be systematic in your further examination, perhaps working from head to toe (a cranio-caudal approach). In tuberous sclerosis there are a multitude of features that you could discuss. You may wish to ask if a UV or Wood's light is available in order to demonstrate hypomelanotic patches more clearly, or offer to perform fundoscopy to identify retinal hamartomas.

Major features of tuberous sclerosis are:

- Facial angiofibromas or forehead plaques
- Periungual fibromas (outgrowth from nail-beds; don't appear until puberty)
- Shagreen patch (an irregular area of connective tissue over the lumbar region)
- Ash leaf patches (hypomelanotic macules, i.e. areas of whiteness)
- Lymphangioleiomyomatosis and/or renal angiomyolipoma
- Cardiac rhabdomyoma (single or multiple; decrease in size with age)
- Multiple retinal nodular hamartomas
- Cortical tuber
- Subependymal nodules
- Subependymal giant cell astrocytoma.

Minor features of tuberous sclerosis are:

- Multiple randomly distributed pits in dental enamel
- Hamartomatous rectal polyps
- Bone cysts
- Gingival fibromas
- Multiple renal cysts
- Non-renal hamartomas
- Retinal achromic patch
- Cerebral white matter radial migration lines
- Skin tags (molluscum fibrosum pendulum).

To show your understanding of how the disease may present with infantile spasms it may be useful to ask the mother how the child was first diagnosed and whether he has suffered with any seizures (present in 65% of cases). It may also show an understanding of the management of the condition if you ask about any extra help he may receive at home or in the classroom in light of special educational needs.

Behavioural and psychiatric problems are common in tuberous sclerosis and often it is this aspect of the condition which causes the most distress to the family. Autistic spectrum disorder occurs in up to 50% of cases, while disruptive behaviour patterns, hyperactivity and attention impairment may be present in up to 60%. A multidisciplinary team approach is necessary for the holistic management of tuberous sclerosis. Family screening and genetic counselling should be offered to the family to discover any other sufferers, and to quantify the risk for future pregnancies.

REMINDER

There are two causative genes for tuberous sclerosis, and each gene may have a variety of mutation types. TSC1 (9q34) encodes the protein hamartin, while the TSC2 (16p13.3) gene encodes the protein tuberin. Tuberin and hamartin interact to provide regulation of the cell cycle. Interestingly, a subgroup of patients have a genetic abnormality spanning the TSC2 gene and the nearby PKD1 gene (encoding polycystin-1) and are found to have severe early-onset polycystic kidney disease.

COMMENTS ON STATION 6

DIAGNOSIS: GROSS DEVELOPMENTAL DELAY (UNDERLYING CAUSE NOT NEEDED)

The developmental station is not designed to test your knowledge of syndromes and rare developmental disorders. You are to show the examiner that you are able to undertake a structured approach to assessing the developmental progress of a child, and then be able to identify any areas of concern.

In this case you have a child with profound developmental delay, including hearing and vision impairment. The tests used for the formal assessment of hearing and vision should be clearly understood as they are key investigations to aid the community paediatrician presented with a child showing developmental delay.

HEARING

The majority of paediatric doctors will not themselves be involved in performing specific audiology tests; however, it is essential to be able to describe the tests available. More importantly, you should know which test is appropriate for the child presented to you. As a crude bedside test you may choose to assess the child's response to a noise or ability to repeat words, but taking a history from the parent is probably the more reliable indicator in a young child. You should be able to describe the following tests and interpret an audiogram.

TESTS FOR INFANTS UNDER 6 MONTHS OF AGE

The Newborn Hearing Screening Programme (NHSP) is introducing hearing tests for all newborn babies in the UK within the first weeks of life.

1. *Oto-acoustic emissions test*: This is the most commonly used newborn screening test. A computer-generated 'click' is played through a small speaker in an earpiece placed in the child's ear. A microphone (also in the earpiece) then listens for a soft echo, detectable if a healthy cochlea is present. The test is analysed by the computer and gives a 'pass/fail' result.

2. *Automated auditory brain stem response test*: This is also a screening test. The child has headphones placed over the ears and three small sensors are attached to the head. The child should be sleeping for the test. The headphones play a series of tones to the child, and a computer analyses the cerebral electrical responses. This tests both cochlear and auditory nerve function. A 'pass/fail' result is reported by the computer.

3. *Auditory brain stem response test*: If the screening test is failed, the child will be referred for this more detailed test. With a similar set-up to the automated test, the audiologist plays a series of sounds of different amplitudes and frequencies through the headphones while the sensors again transfer information to the computer. A record of the brain stem responses at the varying frequencies is provided and gives detailed information about the child's hearing.

TESTS FOR INFANTS 6 MONTHS TO 2½ YEARS OF AGE

1. *The distraction test*: This is often known as the health visitor distraction test or the infant distraction test. It may be performed as a screening test, although it is being phased out with the introduction of newborn hearing screening. It is usually performed when the child is 7–9 months old. It requires two trained staff: the first to sit behind the child and make standardised test noises (such as the Manchester rattle, warbler, Nuffield rattle or a trained voice), varying them in frequency, while the second observes the child's response to the sound. The reliability of this test is improved by it being performed in the audiology clinic. The child must be able to sit unsupported and have good head control.

The following *behavioural tests* are tests involving toys and play techniques in which the child listens for a variety of different sounds as part of a game.

2. *Visual reinforcement audiometry test*:
   - *Loudspeakers:* Specific sounds are played through loudspeakers to the child, who is then observed for a response. On turning to the sound the child will be rewarded by a visual display (the lighting up of a toy or puppet).
   - *Bone conduction:* A vibration is generated through a device placed on each side of the child's head (bypasses middle ear) and the response observed.

- Inserts: Headphones are used instead of loudspeakers. This allows a more accurate assessment of hearing at different frequencies and amplitudes and will allow an audiogram to be produced.

TESTS FOR CHILDREN 2½ YEARS OF AGE AND ABOVE

1. *Speech discrimination test*: The examiner tests the child's ability to hear words at different volume levels without visual information.
2. *Pure tone audiometry test (air and bone conduction)*: An audiometer produces pure sounds at certain frequencies and loudness, or vibrations at certain levels, and the child must respond with a button press or with a movement as part of a game.
3. *Auditory steady-state evoked response test*: This is similar to the automated auditory brain stem response test and involves the analysis of cerebral electrical activity monitored in response to sounds played into the ear by headphones.

VISION

Vision is an important sense that is key to the development of communication skills, orientation and movement, the activities of daily life (ADL) and sustained near-vision tasks like reading and writing. In order to ensure the most appropriate interventions and provision of special educational services, we must assess visual functioning and ability in each of these four areas.

In the examination you may be required to 'examine the eyes' in the neurology or 'other' stations, in which case an assessment of acuity, visual fields, eye movements including squint, pupillary reaction and fundoscopy would be expected. In the developmental station you may wish to approach vision and fine motor development together, aiming to assess the functional application of vision and/or its impairment. For example, by assessing the ability of the child to fix and follow a face, reach for toys or pick up hundreds and thousands from the table you will be able to comment on the visual acuity of the child. If there appears to be significant delay in fine motor skills (as in this case) you should offer a more formal eye examination.

A knowledge of age-appropriate tests and findings is essential (see table opposite). These tests are used as screening tests or as part of an initial examination in those at risk of visual defects. If any abnormality is found, the child should be referred to an ophthalmologist for formal assessment of their vision. In the areas described the child in this question has a global developmental delay with area-specific ages:

- Gross motor: 2–4 months
- Fine motor: 2–4 months
- Vision: significant visual impairment
- Speech, language and hearing: 2–3 months
- Social, emotional and behaviour: 6 weeks.

The key principle with development is to work through a checklist of milestones in your mind and the approximate age of acquisition. If for each

Age	Test or developmental level
Newborn	Check for red reflex (retinoblastoma), cataracts, ptosis, enlarged eyes (glaucoma)
6 weeks	Expected to fix and follow faces/light for 45°
8–12 weeks	Social smile and effective interaction, fix and follow for 180°
6–8 months	Eyes should be aligned, only intermittent brief squint acceptable (e.g. when sleepy); hand regard, hands to mouth, directed reaching and transferring objects
9–11 months	Grip development, recognise family versus strangers from face
1 year	Pick up individual 'hundreds and thousands' (pincer grip)
2–3 years	Preferential looking or picture card tests for visual acuity, cover test for squint
3 years	Sheridan–Gardner test (letter-matching test)
4 years plus	Snellen chart (standardised test of visual acuity)

area of development you can reach a 'passed milestone' and a 'failed milestone' you can then build up an assessment of the child's developmental age and present it to the examiner clearly.

For example, Jimmy was able to do *this* but not yet able to do *that*; therefore his gross motor developmental age is approximately *x* months.

COMMENTS ON STATION 7

It is essential when entering the room to be clear that you are in a role-play and you are to take on the character assigned in the instructions. You will be welcomed in briefly by the examiner and shown to the 'subject', in this case James' mother. You should then introduce yourself clearly to that person.

The following would be appropriate:

'Good morning, my name is Dr X and I am the registrar working with your consultant. Thank you for meeting with me today. Please take a seat. I have made this time available for us to catch up with James' progress and for me to keep you updated on any developments.'

It is polite and shows your understanding of the delicate nature of what you are about to say if you offer the mother the opportunity to call anyone else that she wishes to be present (e.g. her partner).

The topic of MRSA is commonly bandied across the tabloids and broadsheets so most people will have heard and come to an opinion about it. It would therefore be important to mention the word 'MRSA' and then ask what the term meant to the mother.

You could continue by saying that *Staphylococcus aureus* is found to colonise 30% of the general population. MRSA is one type of this bacteria and can also be found on the skin of healthy people in the community, as well as colonising hospital populations. You can link on to talking about how it is routinely tested for when patients transfer from one hospital to another, mentioning those patients then have decontamination treatment of the skin and nose.

It is important to let an aggressive mother have her say. Never interrupt her; simply wait for an opportune break and then perhaps say how you can understand why she might be concerned about such news. You can reassure her that the MRSA bacteria can be treated and that her son is well and will only require topical antibiotics. Remember, you are in an exam and the mother is likely to be played by a hospital worker or paid actress and will have a set agenda. She will also be aware that she must give you an opportunity to talk!

If the mother is using the term 'killer bug' it implies that she is concerned for the life of her child. Be sympathetic; in this case reassurance would be possible. Were you to be given the scenario that James is suffering from MRSA sepsis you may well have to explain what treatments are on offer and that you will of course be monitoring him for any change in his condition.

The mother may ask you, 'Does it mean the tertiary hospital is unclean?'. It would be rather unprofessional and uncharitable to answer this question in the positive! MRSA is a much more ubiquitous organism than it once was. You must make the mother aware of this and how every unit will have a policy for dealing with MRSA. The finding of MRSA does not mean James contracted it there. There are systems in place at all hospitals to prevent spread of infection but you will of course feed this information back to the tertiary hospital.

COMMENTS ON STATION 8

It is important to introduce yourself politely and professionally. You are the registrar in paediatrics and should refer to yourself as 'Dr X'. If you have not been given the name of the mother you should ask it so that you can refer to her easily through the rest of the interview.

The history given suggests that David has had a systemic reaction to the peanut butter with associated wheeze. This would be classed as an anaphylactic reaction in the presence of an atopic family history. Subsequent reactions could be worse and you must be aware of life-threatening features:

- Stridor due to laryngeal and pharyngeal oedema (tongue, lips and uvula)
- Severe bronchospasm
- Hypotension due to systemic vasodilation
- Hypovolaemia (capillary leak).

Generally the management plan would be dependent on the reaction the child had suffered, the feelings of the mother and the services available to your hospital. In this case the APLS management of anaphylaxis needs to be understood. You would grade the severity of any reaction and give adrenaline (epinephrine) (or EpiPen), chlorphenamine, salbutamol and hydrocortisone or methylprednisolone as appropriate.

- *Severe*: Symptoms of airway compromise, shock, neurological signs, or severe gastrointestinal upset
- *Moderate*: Symptoms include respiratory symptoms (breathlessness, wheeze, chest tightness), dizziness, sweating, nausea, vomiting, abdominal pain
- *Mild*: Manifestations are limited to the skin only (urticaria, erythema, angioedema)

For mild reactions an antihistamine may be all that is required. A clear, written plan and adequate provision of the medication would be essential – in this case an EpiPen and training for all those involved in the care of the child. An explanation of life-threatening signs and the importance of calling 999 should be expressed clearly. A MedicAlert bracelet application form may be offered to the family.

The EpiPen (*http://www.epipen.com*) is to be administered when a child has signs or symptoms of anaphylaxis. The dose of adrenaline (epinephrine) is given by the auto-injector through the clothes if necessary. You should follow the 'instructions for use' on the patient information leaflet.

The auto-injector has a grey activation cap and a black tip (the 'needle end'). Once the activation cap is removed, the EpiPen is held with a palmar grasp grip. It is then swung and jabbed firmly against the outer thigh perpendicular to the skin (black tip first). Hold the pen firmly in place for a few seconds, then remove and gently massage the injection area for 10 seconds. Check the needle is visible as this ensures the dose has been administered. Dispose of the EpiPen as instructed and immediately attend the nearest emergency department for medical attention.

In terms of follow-up, it is not unreasonable in a role-play to state that you will arrange for the dietician to see the family immediately after your consultation to discuss peanut avoidance and the allergy specialist nurse to answer any questions that are remaining. You can offer the family a contact number for the allergy nurse and give them a repeat appointment for your allergy clinic.

When trying to show how you successfully transferred information to the mother it is useful to ask her to repeat back to you the key facts that she has understood.

REMINDER

It is easy to use medical terms without thinking when talking to parents. Medical terms can be used but you must then give an explanation of what they mean.

- *Angioedema*: Swelling lips/tongue
- *Stridor*: Noisy breathing
- *Shock*: Pale and lethargic
- *Urticaria*: Severe hives or blotchiness.

The structure of the next 13 minutes is essential in order to cover the necessary topic areas. Below is a proposed approach.

Introduce yourself and ask for the carers' names. It is important to ascertain their relationship to the child. Thank the carers for bringing the child to see you today.

You should get some essential background information, as you would with any new presentation:

- Problem list, teams involved in the child's care
- Past medical or surgical problems
- Medication, allergies, immunisations
- Birth and development
- Social arrangement and allied medical professional involvement
- Family history.

It would then be important to spend the majority of the remaining time taking a clear history of the diet, what concerns the parents and what approaches have already been tried. You may find that they have a suggested management plan from their actual medical team or dietician and they may offer this information to you.

As the bell rings (at 9 minutes in) to give you the last 4 minutes, you might start to summarise the information and, by a systems review, check you have not missed any vital information. You should then give the carers an opportunity to ask you any questions. You can spend some time at the end collecting your thoughts prior to the patient and carers leaving and the examiner beginning the discussion.

In terms of questions relating to diet you will be aiming to find out:

- What is the feed regimen (type of feed, volume, bolus feeds, overnight continuous feed)?
- Any nutritional supplements (e.g. Maxijul®)?
- How is it given?
- Are they giving anything orally?
- Have they kept a food diary?
- Has the child benefited from the gastrostomy?
- How do the carers feel about using the gastrostomy?
- Has the child vomited, had abdominal symptoms or had bowel upset?
- Why is the child more tired? Are they not sleeping?

In a 'failure to thrive' or 'static weight' scenario, you may divide causes into:

- Insufficient energy intake (inappropriate strength or volume feed)
- Inability to absorb feed/components (malabsorption from GI illness, pancreatic insufficiency, feed intolerance or reduced transit time)
- Excessive energy expenditure (coexisting illness, heart failure, sports).

Are there any other co-morbidities making the child have an increased energy expenditure?

What is the weight pattern (plot on the growth chart)?

What factors do the carers feel are responsible for the weight problem?

What do the carers feel should be the next step?

The examiner will have heard the entire history-taking exercise and you should therefore concentrate your presentation on the key diagnoses and current problems. You should summarise what you feel are the factors affecting the diet and weight gain and then give a sensible approach to dealing with these issues. You should not simply relay all the information you have just gained verbatim back to the examiner.

The examiner may raise specific issues with you regarding Rett's syndrome.

Rett's syndrome (RS) is a neurodevelopmental disorder almost exclusively affecting females. Those affected show initially normal development, but later there is a characteristic loss of speech, purposeful hand use and developmental regression. Most cases result from mutations in the MECP2 gene.

The main features of the syndrome include:

- Deceleration of head growth (may be the first sign of Rett's syndrome)
- Stereotypic hand movements (midline hand-wringing, hand-to-mouth movements, licking or repetitive grasping)
- Seizures (variety of types, 50% intractable)
- Autistic features
- Gross motor dysfunction and ataxia
- Abnormal breathing patterns (apnoea and hyperventilation).

The condition tends to progress in stages, with initial developmental arrest (6–18 months) followed by a rapid deterioration and/or regression (1–4 years). The child may then appear to be in a stationary phase until a late motor deterioration (10 years onwards).

Growth failure and malnutrition are important factors in Rett's syndrome. The head circumference, weight and height plots show a tendency to drift from the 50th centile to the 5th centile. This may occur as a result of increased energy expenditure, chronic illness, inadequate nutritional intake or feeding difficulties. Oromotor dysfunction, oesophageal dysmotility and gastro-oesophageal reflux may all be contributing factors in the feeding difficulties seen in Rett's syndrome.

Appendix: Child Development Stages

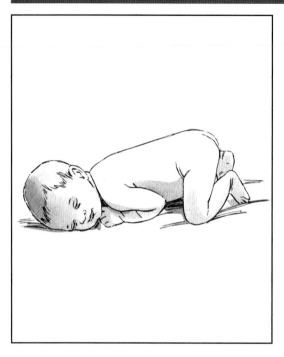

Gross Motor

1. Head up 45–90°
2. Head lag on pull to sit
3. Symmetrical limb movement

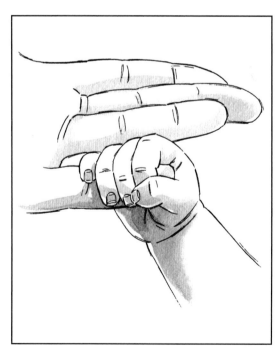

Vision and Fine Motor

1. Follows past midline
2. Grasp reflex
3. Turns toward a light

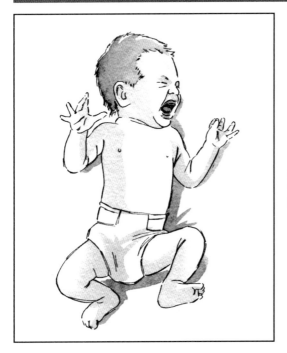

Hearing, Speech and Language

1. Reacts to noise
2. Cries

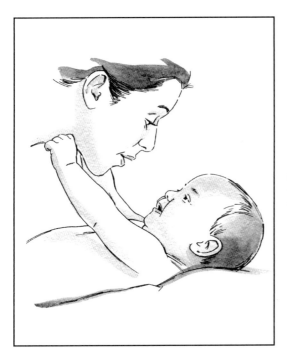

Social, Emotional and Behaviour

1. Recognises primary carer
2. Smiles responsively

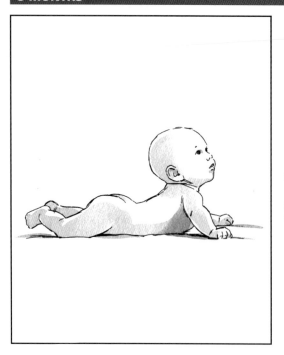

Gross Motor

1. Head steady when sitting supported
2. Lifts head and chest when prone
3. Almost no head lag on pull to sit

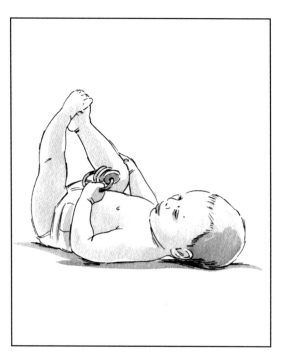

Vision and Fine Motor

1. Follows to 180°
2. Grasps a rattle if placed in hand
3. Plays with hands together

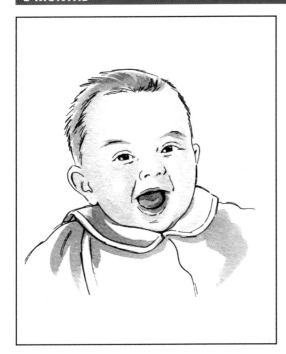

Hearing, Speech and Language

1. Monosyllabic
2. Squeals
3. Turns to a sound
4. Responds to their name being called

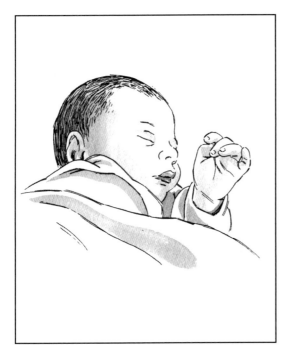

Social, Emotional and Behaviour

1. Smiles spontaneously
2. Laughs
3. Understands cause and effect
4. 70% sleep through the night

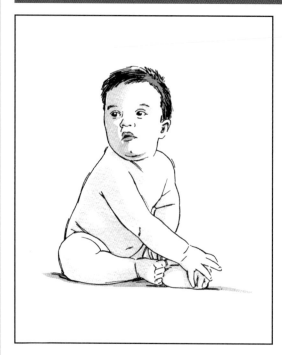

Gross Motor
1. Sits with hunched back or straight back if held
2. Rolls back to front
3. Use their shoulders on pull to sit
4. Can bear almost all their weight
5. Can hold their own feet

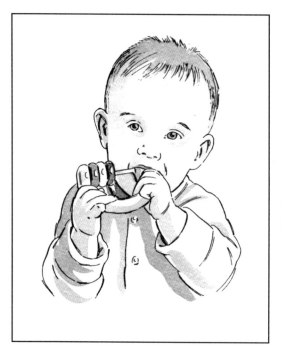

Vision and Fine Motor
1. Palmar grasp
2. Transfers
3. Takes 2 cubes, i.e. doesn't forget 1st
4. Places objects in mouth

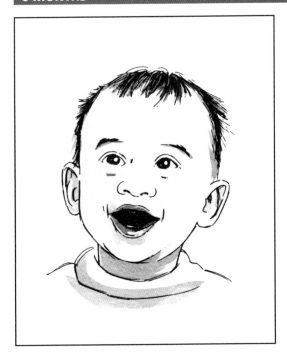

Hearing, Speech and Language

1. Turns to voice
2. Bisyllabic
3. Understands meaning of words
4. Squeals with delight

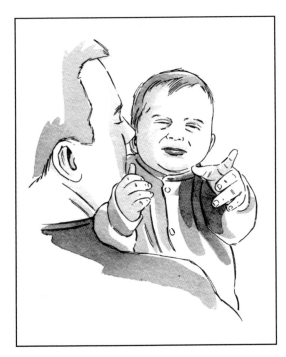

Social, Emotional and Behaviour

1. Tries for a toy out of reach
2. Resists toy pull
3. Not shy with strangers
4. Distress on mother leaving

Circuits for the MRCPCH

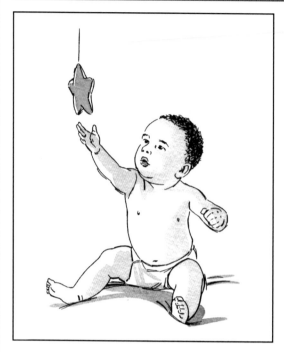

Gross Motor

1. Sits with a straight back
2. Can reach for toy while sitting
   (i.e. able to self–right)
3. Rolls front to back
4. Pulls to stand

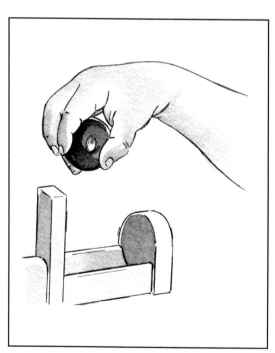

Vision and Fine Motor

1. Pincer grip at 10–12 months
2. Releases toy
3. Bangs 2 cubes together
4. Looks for dropped object

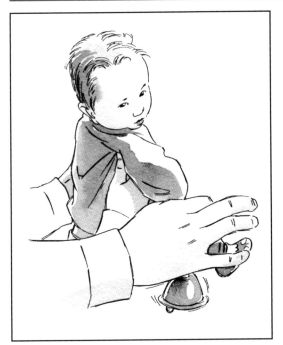

Hearing, Speech and Language

1. 'Mama' or 'Dada'
2. Can perform distraction hearing test

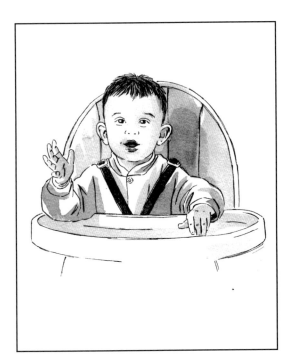

Social, Emotional and Behaviour

1. Plays peek-a-boo
2. Plays alone for long periods
3. Shows likes and dislikes
4. Understands 'No'
5. Waves bye-bye
6. Stranger anxiety

Circuits for the MRCPCH

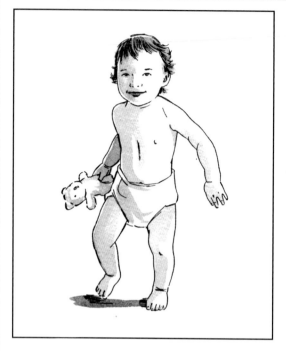

Gross Motor

1. Gets to sitting
2. Gets to stand unaided

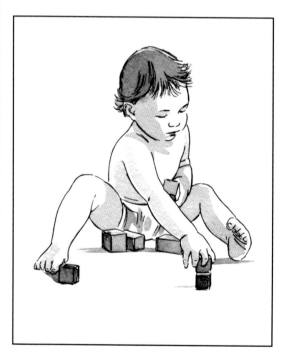

Vision and Fine Motor

1. Turns several pages of a book at once
2. Can see nearly as well as an adult

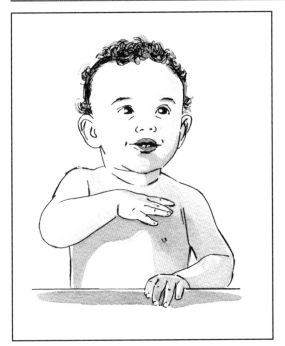

Hearing, Speech and Language

1. 3–5 words
2. Understands instructions

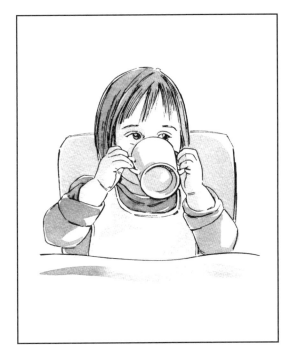

Social, Emotional and Behaviour

1. Plays ball with the examiner
2. Enjoys television
3. Discriminates tastes
4. Looks where someone points
5. Labile moods
6. Still shy with strangers

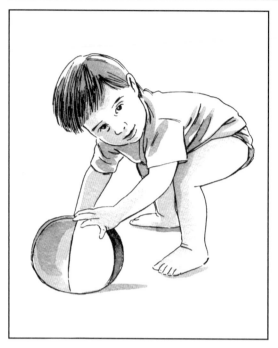

Gross Motor

1. Walks up steps
2. Throws ball overhand
3. Kicks a ball
4. Climbs onto a chair, turns round and sits
5. Squats to pick up a toy
6. Can run steadily but cannot avoid objects
7. Can go up/down stairs with hand held

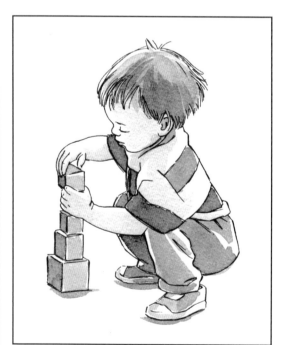

Vision and Fine Motor

1. Tower of 4 blocks
2. Holds a crayon in palm and scribbles
3. Can thread large beads
4. Can remove small object from bottle

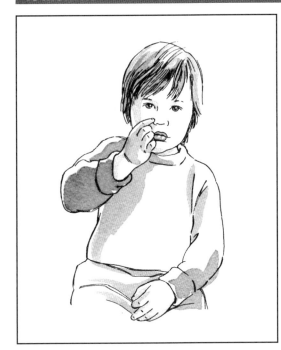

Hearing, Speech and Language

1. Identifies 1–4 body parts
2. Combines words
3. Follows directions
4. Refer to themselves by name

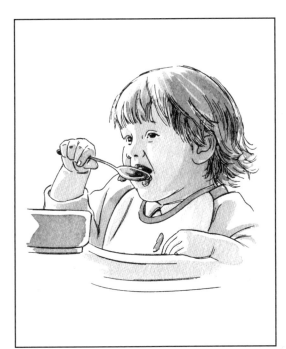

Social, Emotional and Behaviour

1. Will spoon food to mouth
2. Will feed teddy (symbolic play)
3. Helps in house
4. Removes garments
5. Self-recognition in a mirror
6. Remembers where objects belong
7. Eager for independence, e.g. dresses
8. Likes things that screw/unscrew
9. Enjoys posting, stacking, matching, etc.

Circuits for the MRCPCH

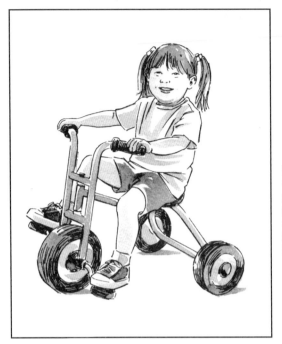

Gross Motor

1. Jumps on the spot
2. Pedals tricycle
3. Runs avoiding obstacles
4. Climbs onto furniture
5. Throws overhand (cannot catch)
6. Walks up/down stairs (both feet/step)

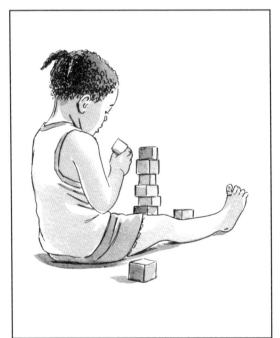

Vision and Fine Motor

1. Tower of 6–8 cubes
2. Imitates vertical line within 30°
3. Draws a circle or dots
4. Turns single pages

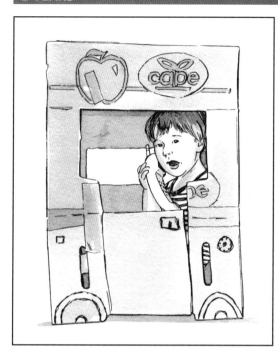

Hearing, Speech and Language
1. Two-word phrase
2. Over 200 words
3. Talk to themselves
4. Plurals

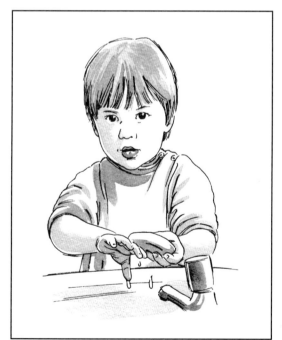

Social, Emotional and Behaviour
1. Dry by day
2. Puts on clothes
3. Washes and dries hands
4. Plays interactive games, e.g. tag
5. Understands consequences, e.g. fall = break
6. Empathic
7. Say how they feel
8. Tantrums as unable to express themselves
9. Dresses and toilets independently
10. Symbolic play

Circuits for the MRCPCH

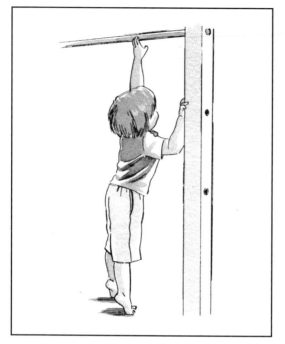

Gross Motor

1. Standing broad jump
2. Stands on tip-toes
3. Kicks a large ball badly

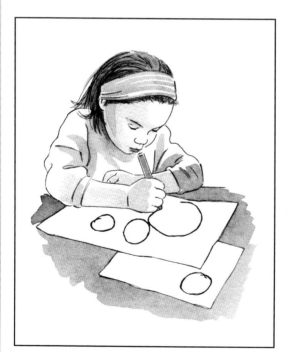

Vision and Fine Motor

1. Copies a circle
2. May use a fork

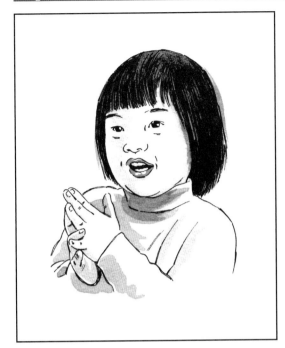

Hearing, Speech and Language

1. Gives first and last name
2. Continually asking questions
3. Uses pronouns correctly (I, me, you)
4. Can say a few nursery rhymes

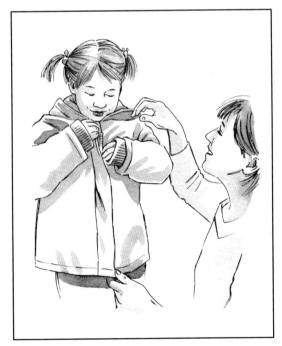

Social, Emotional and Behaviour

1. Separates from mother easily
2. Dresses with supervision
3. Recognise themselves in a photo
4. May be dry at night (large variation)

Circuits for the MRCPCH

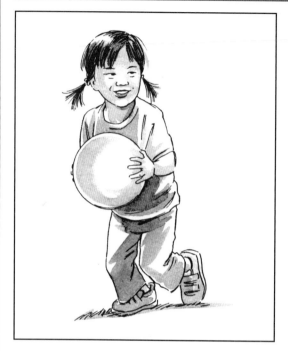

Gross Motor

1. Balances on 1 foot for 1 second
2. Hops on one foot
3. Walks backwards and sideways
4. Up stairs 1 foot per step (2 down)
5. Catches a large ball

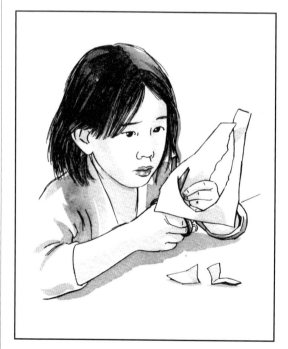

Vision and Fine Motor

1. Copies 'V', 'H' and 'T'
2. Picks the longer line
3. Tower of 8–9 cubes or bridge
4. Pen with thumb and first 2 fingers
5. Cuts paper with scissors
6. Draws a head with legs

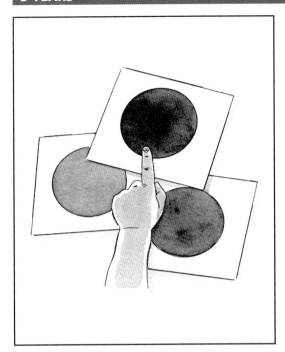

Hearing, Speech and Language

1. Understands 'cold', 'hungry' and 'tired'
2. Counts 1–10 but without knowledge of quantity
3. Does not comprehend above about 3

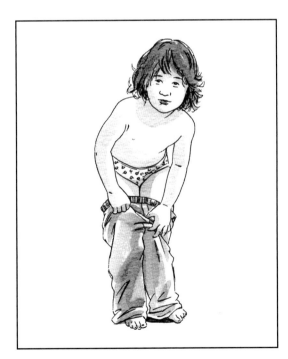

Social, Emotional and Behaviour

1. Dresses without supervision
2. Begins to understand concept of time
3. Interested by cause and effect
4. Develops fears, e.g. the dark
5. Makes friends
6. Aware of gender differences
7. Likes jigsaws

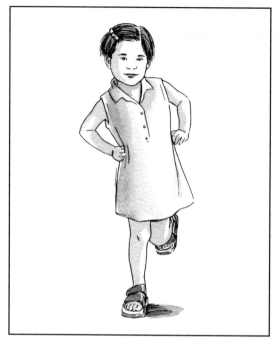

Gross Motor

1. Balances on 1 foot for 5 seconds
2. Catches bounced ball
3. Backward heel-toe
4. Up AND down stairs one at a time
5. Enjoys climbing frames

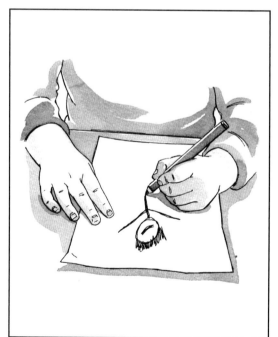

Vision and Fine Motor

1. Draws a man (3–6 parts)
2. Can copy steps using 6 blocks
3. Holds and uses a pencil like an adult
4. Can oppose fingers and thumb in turn
5. Washes and dries hands
6. Cleans teeth
7. Undresses and dresses bar buttons, laces

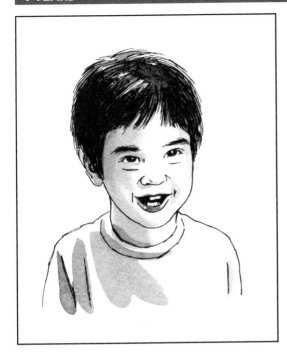

Hearing, Speech and Language

1. Defines words
2. Counts to 20 (understands to 3)
3. Can give reasons
4. Confuses fact and fiction
5. Full name and address
6. Enjoys jokes
7. Patterns, e.g. 'I goed' or 'I runned' because the past tense involved adding-ed

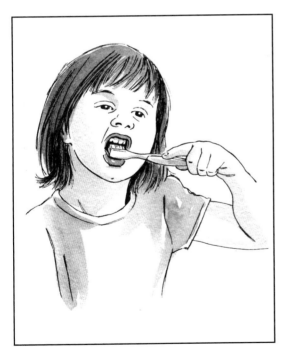

Social, Emotional and Behaviour

1. Will sort objects into groups

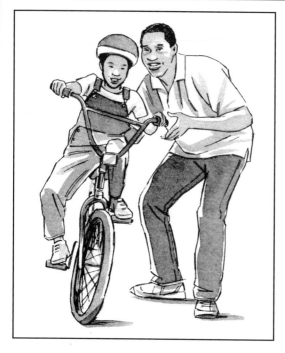

Gross Motor

1. Begins to ride bike without stabilisers
2. Touches toes without bending knees
3. Hops and skips

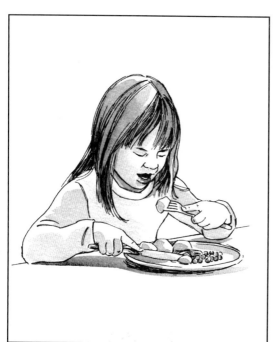

Vision and Fine Motor

1. Uses knife and fork competently
2. Draws head, body, legs, nose, mouth and eyes
3. Copies 4 steps with 10 cubes
4. Copies a square but not a triangle

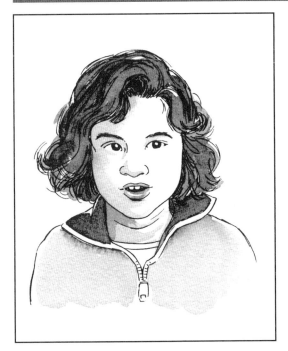

Hearing, Speech and Language

1. Name, age, address and birthday
2. Fluent speech and grammatically correct

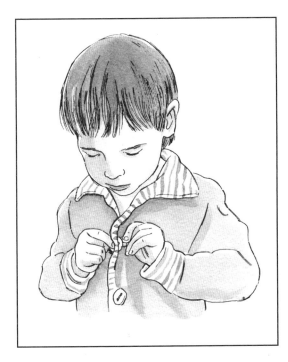

Social, Emotional and Behaviour

1. Choose their own friends
2. Very definite likes/dislikes, e.g. carrots in strips, not rounds
3. Buttons up
4. Amuse themselves for long periods

Index